The Social Life of Health Data

Alena Thiel · Samuel Aniegye Ntewusu
Editors

The Social Life of Health Data

Health Records and Knowledge Production in Ghana

palgrave
macmillan

Editors
Alena Thiel
Department of Social Anthropology
Martin-Luther-Universität
Halle-Wittenberg
Halle (Saale), Germany

Samuel Aniegye Ntewusu
Institute of African Studies
University of Ghana
Accra, Ghana

ISBN 978-981-97-3499-3 ISBN 978-981-97-3500-6 (eBook)
https://doi.org/10.1007/978-981-97-3500-6

This Palgrave Macmillan imprint is published by the registered company Springer Nature Singapore Pte Ltd.
The registered company address is: 152 Beach Road, #21-01/04 Gateway East, Singapore 189721, Singapore

Acknowledgements

The idea for this book originated at a workshop held in Accra in 2022, which brought together scholars working on broad issues relating to health and the production of health records in Ghana. Our vibrant discussions around issues of the evolution of the standardising force of health registration throughout Ghanaian history and its varying encounters with medical pluralism have inspired the collection of arguments in this book. We are grateful for the participants who shared their insights and critical readings of early drafts of the papers, and appreciate their patience and continued commitment to this project through several rounds of reviews and revisions.

Alena Thiel gratefully acknowledges support from the German Research Foundation (Grant TH2432/2-1) for funding the workshop and publication of this book.

Contents

Notes on Contributors

Humphrey Asamoah Agyekum is an Assistant Professor at the Centre for Global Criminology at the Department of Anthropology, University of Copenhagen. His research interests range from security to mental health. He has published on mental health among Ghanaian youth. His monograph is titled *From Bullies to Officers and Gentlemen: How Notions of Professionalism and Civility Transformed the Ghana Armed Forces*.

Florence Naab is an Associate Professor of infertility and psychosocial health. She is the Dean of the University of Ghana School of Nursing and Midwifery. She is an expert in the area of psychosocial health problems associated with infertility. She has completed research projects on male infertility, female infertility, and the relationship between the beliefs that women hold about being infertile and their psychosocial health problems. She has investigated the levels of depression, anxiety, stigma, stress, and social isolation among women with infertility.

Diana Amoni Ntewusu is a Medical Sociologist with a Ph.D. from the University of Ghana, Legon. Her research interests are in the Sociology of Health, Illness and Health Care; Health Services Administration; and Indigenous Knowledge Systems. She currently works as a Research Scientist with the Science and Technology Policy Research Institute—Council for Scientific and Industrial Research (CSIR—STEPRI), Accra, Ghana.

Samuel Aniegye Ntewusu is the Director of the Institute of African Studies, University of Ghana. He has promoted historical studies at the graduate level by researching and teaching courses related to Historiography and Methodology, Africa's Colonial and post-independence history, The Slave Trade and Africa, and Pan-Africanism, among others. He has developed an undergraduate course on Chieftaincy and Development with a focus on the role of chiefs in economic and democratic governance in Africa. He has produced several articles and book chapters, a monograph on Urban and Transport History, and co-edited a book on aspects of History, Gender, and Culture in Africa and Europe.

Lillian Akorfa Ohene is a Senior Lecturer and Head of the Department for Public Health Nursing, School of Nursing and Midwifery, University of Ghana. She is a certified pediatric nurse who holds a Ph.D. in Nursing. Dr. Ohene has over eighteen years of practice and teaching experience in higher academic institutions. Her research focuses on the holistic care of sick children and the well-being of women and their families. As a qualitative researcher, Dr. Ohene has extensively explored the well-being of families of patients with acute and chronic conditions in hospitals. She has also contributed to developing nursing and midwifery knowledge in Ghana.

Vivian Efua Senoo-Dogbey is a Lecturer at the Public Health Department of the School of Nursing and Midwifery, University of Ghana, Legon. She has dedicated her research efforts to understanding Health Care Worker's infection prevention and safety behaviour and practices against blood-borne infectious diseases which could be occupationally acquired. Dr. Senoo-Dogbey has investigated healthcare workers' infection prevention practices, specifically vaccination practices, post-exposure prophylaxis uses and practices, serological testing, and antibody levels. Her works also focus on the preventive behaviour of women and families regarding the vertical transmission of hepatitis B virus infection.

Oliver Kofi Tasin is a tutor at the Social Sciences Department of St. Francis College of Education, Hohoe, and a Ph.D. Candidate in the Department of History and Diplomacy at the University of Cape Coast, Ghana. His research interest focuses on the social history of Ghana, specifically colonial and post-colonial medical practices in northern Ghana.

Alena Thiel is a social anthropologist with over a decade of research experience in Ghana. Her recent work covers public sector digitalisation, statistical production, and the development of information systems, with a particular focus on health data. She is the PI of the project "How Democracies Know: Identification Technologies and Quantitative Analyses of Development in Ghana" (German Research Foundation, 2019–2023), and affiliated Senior Researcher in the project "African Technoscapes" as well as in the Law, Organisation, Science and Technology research group (LOST).

List of Figures

CHAPTER 1

Developing an Interdisciplinary Reading of Ghanaian Health Data Histories: An Introduction

Samuel Aniegye Ntewusu and Alena Thiel

1.1 Introduction

Health data is indispensable for the routine operation, monitoring, and planning of interventions in public health systems. Within population data ecosystems at large, administrative health registers are often among the most sophisticated systems, as the "ability to measure and monitor the health of populations" in terms of epidemiology, demography, and biostatistics is a prerequisite for public health decision-making (AbouZahr & Boerma, 2005). Ghana's health information system in particular has attracted intensive foreign donor attention, fuelling investments in infrastructure and capacity. These investments, however, are

S. A. Ntewusu
University of Ghana, Accra, Ghana
e-mail: santewusu@ug.edu.gh

A. Thiel (✉)
Martin-Luther-University Halle-Wittenberg, Halle, Germany
e-mail: alena.thiel@ethnologie.uni-halle.de

A. Thiel and S. A. Ntewusu (eds.), *The Social Life of Health Data*,
https://doi.org/10.1007/978-981-97-3500-6_1

often made without much critical interrogation of the proliferation of multiple (and at times competing) infrastructures, platforms, and standards (Erikson, 2012), or their far-reaching impacts on Ghanaians' lives—for example, as seen across the globe in the restrictions in mobility accompanying the drive for real-time monitoring of the Covid-19 pandemic (Ntewusu, 2020; Thiel & Agyekum, 2023). The present volume was inspired by a collection of researchers interested in various aspects of Ghana's health system, and by the observation that practices of recording health in Ghana's colonial past and the country's present-day health system have remained understudied. The present volume seeks to address this gap by detailing from multiple disciplinary angles the procedures through which Ghanaian health professionals organise knowledge about health, and how these practices are both conditioned by larger societal developments while at the same time "retroactively" (Desrosières, 2015) impacting Ghanaian society.

Zooming in from different disciplinary angles, we position health-related knowledge practices—whether oral, written, or digital—as central to the maintenance of colonial and contemporary power relations. We also show that the forces of standardisation at various moments of Ghana's history have co-opted plural medical practice in diverse ways, e.g. in the capture of oral traditional knowledge by colonial medical officers for the treatment of tropical diseases, or in the professionalisation of traditional medical practice through the mobilisation of quantitative forms of evidence. Hence, the case studies in this volume paint a complex picture of how standardisation and medical pluralism interact in practice.

Where the literature has presented the diversity of health data production in Ghana and other developing countries, it generally foregrounded the issue of access to basic health care in the context of low penetration of health services. For example, studies on telecommunication and health care have covered the remote provision of midwifery, advice services, and verbal autopsies (Al Dahdah et al., 2015; Duclos, 2015). Information Systems research on the other hand has given intensive attention to the genealogy, setup, and operation of Health Information Management Systems (Gyaase & Bright, 2019; Miscione & Staring, 2009; Sæbø et al., 2011); the digital labour required to populate such registers (Siyam et al., 2021); the participation of private sector innovations (Burchardt & Umlauf, 2023); and other forms of non-clinical institutions in the datafication of health (Feldman et al., 2018; Ruckenstein & Schüll, 2017). However, little attention has been paid to registration practices and "the ways that data technology enables or constrains human experience" (Ruckenstein & Schüll, 2017, p. 271). This is highly problematic, as "[p]opulations do not simply exist as objects of knowledge, but are products of data practices" and "particular technologies of counting and modelling" (Hoeyer et al., 2019, pp. 462, 466). For this reason, our argument departs from recent studies of health information systems that have predominantly focused on management practices. Instead, we seek to contribute to the field our observations around the social dimensions of health data practices. Scholars who have adopted critical social science approaches have certainly advanced the debate around international efforts to impose global health standards (e.g. as explored by Patterson, 2018; Prince, 2014) and the particular role of metricisation therein (Adam, 2016). Biruk's *Cooking Data: Culture and Politics in an African Research World* (2018) particularly serves as an inspiration for detailing in a thick, qualitative manner both the global interconnections and local situatedness of data practices in a single country case, in this case Malawi. We take inspiration from Biruk when zooming in on the case of Ghana to describe at proximity the expert knowledges, materialities, and implications of health data collection across historical periods and shifting socio-political alignments. In distinction to Biruk, we go beyond the level of global health research and instead open our investigation to the micro-processes in the Ghanaian health data system at large, along with specific attention to its infrastructural arrangements, and the convergence of several materialities, or types of registers, participating in the constitution of composite health realities.

Before elaborating the critical advancements made by the contributors to this volume, we deem it necessary to clarify how we conceptualise the multiple knowledge practices that accompany the varying interventions in health that are presented in this volume.

1.2 Health Data, Knowledge, Information: Defining the Concepts

The arguments presented in this volume differentiate between the terms health information, health data, knowledge production, and registration practices. Hence a word regarding definition is in order. Specifically, when we talk about information, we follow Harold Garfinkel's sociological theory of information (Garfinkel, 2008). Here, information is characterised, first, by its actual, rather than merely conceptual properties (Rawls, 2008, pp. 45, 46). It must, in other words, be transformable and able to be "stored, owned, lost and found" (Rawls, 2008, p. 46). Different from knowledge, which is widely shared, information is distributed unevenly across populations and must therefore be allowed a degree of incompleteness, ambiguity, and even "ignorance" (Rawls, 2008: 46). Garfinkel's theory is particularly relevant to our present argument, as it draws our attention to the social nature of information. To be intelligible, information manifests itself as a clear order of symbols, signals, and messages by "those actors who are engaged in a situation together and committed to a shared practice (…) There is no information without an order generated by actors orienting towards rules—or constitutive practices—that they use to produce that order" (Rawls, 2008, p. 47).

Similar to information, data too is profoundly relational in its nature. If information is only meaningful in the context of agreed upon orders, the concept of data points us to "the raw material produced by abstracting the world into categories, measures and other representational forms—numbers, characters, symbols, images, sounds, electromagnetic waves, bits—that constitute the building blocks from which information and knowledge are created" (Kitchin, 2014, p. 1). To describe the nature of data, Kitchin (2014, pp. 4–9) differentiates between data's form (text, images, etc.), organisation (structured, semi-structured, unstructured), and kind (indexical, attribute data, metadata), among other dimensions. For our purposes, it suffices to understand data production as a social activity geared towards some form of value generation, e.g. with the aim to further abstraction, reproducibility, efficiency, and rationalisation, but possibly also political values such as those tied to the process of territorialisation.

Data practices, then, signify the combined practices involved in the production of data for various types of intervention. This includes the "selecting, formatting, editing, storing, cleaning," but also the "standardisation, and classification, as well as the development of methods for retrieval, analysis, visualization, and quality control" of data (Ruppert & Scheel, 2021, pp. 30, 31). Data practices hinge on diverse assemblages of material technologies, as well as methods, expertise, and forms of organisation. At the same time, they entail distinct logics, struggles, and contestations, but also hopes, trust, and claims to legitimacy, truth, and validity (Ruppert & Scheel, 2019, p. 234). This is relevant as, oftentimes, data practices support the logic of testing, which

> has become a critical practice to know unknowns, identify risks, and orient actions at a time when often interpretations of the evidence base rather than the political imaginary of a better world generate legitimacy for policy decisions. Sometimes, however, experimenting, testing, and measuring produce disorienting results that do nothing to resolve a situation. (Beisel et al., 2018, p. 109)

We concur with these authors' analysis that testing represents an effort "to make the world more predictable," while also silencing the limits of the test. "[A]s a technique of knowing, it limits itself to comparing a current situation to a standard that was established in advance," while necessarily hiding this assumption to achieve universal applicability (Beisel et al., 2018, p. 109).

Positing health information, knowledge, and data as fundamentally social phenomena that performatively hide their world-making impact requires us to explore them in light of their specific contexts of production. Here, the focus on the work of health registration, or the writing of health, provides us with a useful conceptual avenue. Specifically, we follow anthropologist Susan Reynolds Whyte (2011, pp. 34, 30), who notes that writing is an "integral part of healthcare" that "opens relational possibilities for those who write and those who are written." At the heart of this is the production of "data and treatises that abstract and objectify that knowledge" as it is written into material form, transmitted, and disseminated, while also creating "a more lasting artefact, a medical record that is both a history and a time line into the future" (ibid., p. 36). Whyte's argument not least points us to the authority of written knowledge over other forms of knowing—which is an observation that is central to our case studies as well—and its "capacity to mediate such relations" of power between government and communities while engaging with multiple publics in the "therapeutic marketplace" (Whyte, 2014).

In this edited volume, we propose using the term health registration in a broad fashion, as any measure to contain, in a systematic manner, data on patients and health-related events. Health registration "unfolds on a number of different scales and registers, including data-driven medical research and public health infrastructures, clinical health care, and self-care practices" (Ruckenstein & Schüll, 2017, p. 216; cf. Feldman et al., 2018). Health registration practices, as Sund et al. (2014) have shown, further differ widely in coverage (varying from a total registration to a population sample and from national to regional or local coverage); modes of data collection (such as data collected for various reasons, from economic and administrative purposes to more strict epidemiological purposes); methodology (e.g., registration by the health services or by interviews with patients or population groups); and temporal dimensions (with data being collected continuously or repeatedly with some time intervals). Additionally, we here refer to historically varying types of data and explicitly seek to foreground the material and techno-political shifts that accompany and embed health registration practices at various moment in Ghanaian history. In so doing, we seek to shed particular light on the intersection of materialities of knowledge, the standardisation of health data, and plural medical practice.

1.3 Between Standard and Practice: Medical Pluralism in Interdisciplinary Perspective

Central to our argument is the contributors' common observation that practices of recording health seek to impose (often implicit) standards. Among these forces of standardisation, Erikson (2012, p. 368) has identified the central role of the global health business, along with its administrative structures and technological means of collecting increasing amounts of data. Besides this central vector, the contributors to this book expand our view of the forces of standardisation, foregrounding, among other vectors, an early interest in global health during colonial times (see Tasin, Chapter 2 in this volume). Health standards further originate from international best practices in disease control and prevention, such as standard case definitions and data standards in health reporting. Upon their translation into Ghanaian contexts, these standards encounter plural medical practices, knowledges, and relations of care. Medical pluralism here is understood as the coexistence of multiple conceptions of health and healing, as well as the recognition of their embeddedness within specific socio-technical settings. The chapters in this volume reject the notion that Ghanaian medical professionals blindly submit to globally circulating registration tools and formats. Instead, they illustrate these experts' attunement to, and translation and localisation of standards into the Ghanaian realities. The contributions to this volume present arguments about how different assemblages of health registration—that is, forms of measurement and testing, oral and written practices of retaining information, and the arrangements of data infrastructures, personnel, and expert knowledges at the core of these registration practices—are mobilised and adapted to diverse ends.

In the interest of attuning to the plurality of actors, infrastructures, and practices of health registration, we train an interdisciplinary lens onto the question of how Ghana has generated an apparatus for capturing knowledge about health since colonial times, and how these processes have come to intersect with other clinical and societal transformations, such as the development of ideas of global health, or the ongoing digitalisation of health interventions. Our argument joins perspectives from history, medical anthropology, public health, as well as anthropology, to investigate the layered nature of knowledge infrastructures in Ghana's health domain. The value of such an interdisciplinary approach to knowledge practices is that it probes, from different analytical entry points, into the phenomenon of health registration, and hence allows us to connect its "living" "material," and "technical" elements (Duclos, 2015). Yet, interdisciplinarity also implies "a variety of boundary transgressions," requiring us to transcend deeply internalised "rules, subjectivities and knowledge corpuses" (Barry and Born 2014, p. 1). Despite their varying perspectives, the chapters in this volume align not only through their focus on a common country case, but crucially also through the common goal of providing thick empirical contextualisations of the observed knowledge practices.

We bring together analyses of oral, written, and digital forms of inscription to present a more encompassing account of how experts and professionals—ranging from colonial health officers to contemporary medical practitioners, health policy planners, CSOs, and patient organisations—have established an apparatus for data collection regarding health, throughout Ghana's history. Our first analytical angle is rooted in the historical method. The book's commitment to present the genealogies of health registration taps into well-established descriptions of the key trends in the historical transformations in public health provision. Prince (2014) describes the shifts from early attempts of colonial administrations to improve public health to the post-Independence, developmentalist vision of government-controlled universal healthcare access, and more recently, the rise of private, nongovernmental, and humanitarian service provision following the structural adjustment period in the 1980s. Health care and health data "in colonial Africa was intimately tied to a repressive, coercive, and violent system of power and knowledge, which reached deep into

African lives and identities" under the banner of "modernising" indigenous healing practices (Prince, 2014, p. 4). In this book, we pay specific attention to the infrastructural assemblages, e.g. in connection with transport systems, that contributed to proto-health care in the Gold Coast colony's economy. For example, Ntewusu (Chapter 3 in this volume) highlights the role of motorised and non-motorised means of transport in the context of the transport section of the Medical Field Units (MFUs). They comprised quite a big category in the health delivery system in colonial times, since the activities of the MFU required the movement of personnel and goods. Three modes of transport were utilised in this regard: head portage-carriers, cycle-based transport (bicycles and motorbikes), and motor vehicles. Specifically, the book shows how such arrangements exerted significant control over mobility and economic activities beyond purely clinical applications, while forging complex relations with indigenous medical knowledges, with relations oscillating between suppression, appropriation, and resistance, but also some forms of integrating plural medical approaches. Here, Tasin's (Chapter 2 in this volume) analysis of colonial health policies, particularly policies relating to sleeping sickness, in northern Ghana from 1902 to 1945, shows how colonial concepts of health and medical practice captured indigenous knowledges of health conditions, diagnoses, and treatments. The capture of such knowledge was considered crucial in controlling medical conditions in the Northern Territories, as well as colonial control over this area at large.

The historical chapters by Ntewusu and Tasin highlight the role of the archive in the social construction of reality. Through analysis of archival records, the two chapters not only articulate the processes and practices related to health delivery in the past. They also point to the relevance of studying the processes of transmission of knowledge regarding health systems, and what kinds of knowledges eventually enter the historical record. These questions not least serve as a critical reminder to interrogate the performative nature of health registration in the present as well, as the rest of the chapters reveal.

As already noted, in addition to our close historiographic reading of the interactions of indigenous and colonial ways of organising knowledge around health, the contributors to this book mobilise sociological and anthropological perspectives to explore contemporary ways in which Ghanaian medical professionals are mobilised or potentially demobilised by the standards, methods, and calculative devices that accompany the increasing production of global health data. We connect our historical and contemporary sociological observations by tracing the echoes of the legacies of colonial relations of power in present-day knowledge production. In doing so, the contributors engage closely with the question of the origins of knowledge standards, and how they are folded into relations of power. For example, Amoni's chapter provides a detailed analysis of the legitimating force of quantification in the effort to formalise herbal medical practice in Ghana since early post-Independence time. Her work connects historical dimensions with a contemporary sociological view into the organisation of the association of herbal medical practitioners, showing how they adopt registers of quantification to establish themselves as a professional body.

Combining similar sociological insights into the organisation of HBV preventive practices, and their combination with a distinct public health lens, Senoo-Dogbey, Naab, and Akorfa Ohene lead us into the details of public health best practices and the multiple challenges of their implementation in the Ghanaian clinical context. They point us to the complex interplay of moments of standardisation at the levels of institutional and individual preventive practice, and the challenges of implementing standards in view of infrastructural and funding constraints. Agyekum recasts the question of professional organisation of standards by adopting an anthropological perspective on how forces of standardisation affect the ways mental health patients and their care givers understand psychiatric diagnoses and the social stigma attached to them. He reminds us of the transformative potential of standards, which equip Ghanaian mental health professionals with the means to challenge harmful societal attitudes and practices related to mental health and illness. Zooming in on digital transformations, Thiel finally bookends the empirical chapters, illustrating the unintended desynchronising effects of digitalisation, e.g. when public health professionals navigate the loss of valuable historical data in the trade-off for real-time data storage, in the turn to digital health information management systems.

Taken together, our cases and approaches are positioned within both clinical and regulatory contexts, as well as grounded in the experiences of patients and care givers. Weaving together these various angles, we seek to present in this volume a deeply contextualised account of how travelling models of health (and the standards and blueprints that accompany them, cf. Behrends et al., 2014) impact the construction of illness, healing, and care relations in Ghana's plural medical context. Besides contributing to the interdisciplinary theoretical perspectives of the book, the contributors to this volume each base their analysis on a close qualitative engagement within their distinct fields. Their detailed ethnographic and historiographic work provides us with qualitative insights into the interaction of different actors (including health practitioners, data scientists, and medical committees, but also colonial health officers) with specific knowledge practices and infrastructures. They show how standardisation and medical pluralism intersect, with unexpected effects on the social relations of illness, healing, and care.

1.4 Structure of the Book

The book is structured into three sections, each exploring a particular set of questions on health knowledge practices. Section I, "Health Data Histories," illustrates the important contribution made by the historiographic documentation of health records. Historical approaches construct a knowledge base that offers insights into past regimes' justifications for producing patient records, the nature of such records, and their geographic extent. A proper appreciation of the kind of information collected in historical health records contributes to discourses on the medical history of Ghana, especially regarding the relationship between health and social policies, but also economic development. As Adu-Gyamfi and Oware (2019, p. 18) argue, health policies adopted by the British colonial government were extended to the local people to help improve their health statuses for economic gain. The book goes beyond this observation, using historical health records as a way of reconstructing the creation of the medical world in the present (Warner, 1999). Specifically, adopting the lens of the health register and the production of medical knowledge allows us to illustrate the relationship between medical ideology and medical practice.

Oliver Tasin's chapter opens the collection, choosing as its entry point the attempt at building transnational health interventions in colonial times. Tasin crucially describes indigenous channels of keeping information on health events, and the colonial ambition of integrating these knowledges into standardised records as a form of bringing about State power. The chapter specifically examines colonial campaigns against epidemics and diseases in northern Ghana during the first half of the twentieth century. The Northern Territories of the Gold Coast, or what constitutes today northern Ghana, came under British colonial rule in

1902. In addition to its lack of exportable colonial resources, northern Ghana had the added misfortune of being a locus of many hyper-endemic diseases including yaws, malaria, onchocerciasis, cerebrospinal meningitis, and sleeping sickness. In the 1920s, diseases caused extensive mortality in many communities across the Northern Territories, which had a shattering impact on the southwards labour supply for the Gold Coast's mines and cocoa farms. In response, the administration invested in short-term control measures against the outbreak, while more expansive efforts were directed towards a campaign against the diseases and their vectors. Examining the origins and actual implementation of these measures, the chapter analyses the indigenous and colonial knowledges, strategies, and experiments employed to control diseases. By focusing on the first half of the twentieth century, the study reveals not only the wider patterns of colonial public health policies, but also shows how disease control was integral to the colonial project of economic exploitation and social control. Through the qualitative method of historical research and the use of oral, archival, and secondary sources, the chapter suggests that the colonial administration's public health policies present a viable window for understanding a range of colonial issues, from purely medical ones to political and economic issues. With its specific regional focus, Tasin's chapter provides us with an analysis of the dual health systems in northern Ghana at the time of colonial rule. What is revealing in this chapter is how Britain intensified the administration of Western medicine in the northern part of the country in the years immediately following the Second World War. Tasin ascribes this to an economic interest rather than a desire to provide health care. The chapter contends that it was as a result of the need to kick-start a slowed economy—a factor or trend which was symptomatic of the global system, due to the world war—that made the British intensify healthcare provision to secure a healthy labour force for the purposes of production.

Following Tasin, Samuel Ntewusu's chapter provides fine-grained historical detail on the operation of colonial health and health registration. Focusing on the establishment of the Medical Field Units in the 1930s and 1940s, Ntewusu documents one of the early stages of generating statistical data on populations in what is today the territory of Ghana. Adding to Tasin's discussion of the colonial imprint on Ghana's health system, Ntewusu's chapter provides detailed insights into the operation of healthcare provision, but also into its documentation. The MFUs were established in the 1930s as part of the colonial administration's policy to handle endemic and epidemic diseases. Beginning with a few locations in

Gambaga in northern Ghana, their activities spread to several parts of the country. The MFU represented specialised units in the medical system responsible for epidemics and the treatment of other critical diseases such as yaws, sleeping sickness, malaria, and others. From about 1904, the British colonial administration was extended from the coastal region to include Ashanti and the northern part of Ghana. Referred to as the Northern Territories, that area became the incubator where the MFUs were established. Due to the frequency of outbreak of diseases, small groups of the medical staff moved to specific communities and set up special sites to provide health services. An added role was for them to generate statistical information on diseases and epidemics. With the introduction of technological tools and testing kits, health information was recorded, stored, and shared, and specific trends of diseases were established. Since the activities of the MFU stretched from the northern to the middle belts of Ghana such as Kintampo, and further to Ashanti region, the MFU recorded a picture of the complex nature of epidemics in Ghana. For this reason, the establishment of Medical Field Units marked a critical moment in Ghana's medical history. Prior to the MFU, health delivery and epidemics were handled by means of experimentation, using ad hoc measures. Such ad hoc processes were transformed into a more coordinated process where a wide range of medical staff—junior, senior, technicians, typists, drivers, and many more, distributed in different parts of northern and the middle belt of Ghana—helped track down infections and epidemics. From the demographics presented in the chapter, it is apparent that the operations of the MFU enabled the detection and treatment of more diseases in human populations that were scattered in a manner that otherwise would have made them difficult to track and treat. The chapter points to the significant influence of the MFU in Ghana's health system, as rural communities were greatly impacted by their operations. It traces the origin and operation of the MFU with specific reference to the areas, communities, and populations targeted, and the specific diseases that were treated; examples of these include sleeping sickness, meningitis, smallpox, malaria, and yellow fever. Specific attention is given to the role of infrastructures, such as the staff and transport systems associated with the Medical Field Units, and the problems faced by the personnel in their contribution to recording disease.

Section II of the book, "Ethnographies of the Health Register," investigates contemporary health registration practices from the perspective of medical anthropology and its contextual approaches to understanding health, illness, and healing practices in specific political, economic and socio-cultural settings (Kleinman & Benson, 2006). Our common country case of Ghana has often been described as an environment marked by incomplete public health infrastructure, where common care practices draw together practitioners from clinical institutions, traditional healers, social support, and religious leaders. Across these institutions, diverse forms of recording illness condition experiences of help-seeking, treatment, care relations, as well as the social stigma attached to certain illnesses (Akyeampong, 2015; Akyeampong et al., 2015; Csordas & Lewton, 1998). Section II explores the tensions arising from the health register's attempt at standardising diagnoses in the Ghanaian context of medical pluralism. We situate these tensions in the contemporary moment of the "transfiguration" of (global) health (Kehr et al., 2018), and the increasingly complex flows of data that emerge along with new post-colonial health data politics. The contributors' critical anthropological examination uncovers how knowledge practices are mediated along these data journeys, and with what retroactive effects on the provision of care.

Agyekum explores the effects of the international standardisation of mental health diagnoses on social inscriptions of these issues, especially stigmas associated with mental illness and treatment. Mental health in Ghana has always been a contentious issue due to its association with supernatural forces, such as witchcraft. This has led to mental health being poorly understood as a condition that can be dealt with through the healthcare system. However, in recent years, there seems to have been a change in mental health perceptions in Ghana, driven by both Ghanaian and foreign-trained mental health practitioners. These practitioners are pushing the standardisation of treatment through the application of the Diagnostic and Statistical Manual of Mental Disorders, Fifth Edition, Text Revision (DSM-5-TR), in their professional practices. Based on qualitative methods and ethnographic interviews with Ghanaian mental health experts, Agyekum examines the tensions arising between plural medical views on mental health, that is in standardised registers and in local beliefs and demands. The chapter illuminates the mediating force of the DSM-5-TR, and its effect on the ways in which Ghanaian mental health practitioners apply their knowledge and expertise in a society that considers mental health challenges to belong to the supernatural realm. Agyekum adds to our interrogation of writing practices in healthcare contexts a deep, socio-technically informed reading of the participation of global standards in mental health professional practices.

Located at the intersection of medical anthropology and sociology, the chapter by Diana Amoni takes registration practices as a starting point to analyse how herbal medical practitioners mobilise registers of quantification to establish themselves as a professional body. Traditional medical knowledge has remained important to indigenous populations. In Ghana, the practice has proven to be resilient and creative in the wake of the standardisation of health care emphasised by State policies, and the establishment of formal regulatory institutions. These have led to a kind of medical professionalism, which hitherto was alien to traditional medical practice in Ghana. Amoni's chapter explores the production of statistics on traditional medicine practitioners and their practices and products in Ghana, and how these quantifications participate in professionalising the practice. Drawing on findings from qualitative interviews, and documents provided by the Traditional and Alternative Medicine Directorate, the Traditional Medicine Practice Council, the Food and Drugs Authority, the Centre for Plant Medicine Research, and other relevant stakeholders in the industry, the chapter contributes in-depth descriptions of the standardising procedures devised to professionalise practitioners, their practices, and their products. The chapter concludes that there is no way one can understand traditional medical practice in Ghana without recourse to the statistics generated through regulatory standardising procedures, and the effects of these standards on practitioners, practices, and products, emphasising the co-production of various forms of knowledge and health practices.

Section III, "Health records and the politics of standardisation," finally, explores health data practices in relation to regulation and governance of health. Existing studies of health registration have as their point of departure the production of evidence-based health interventions. Scholarly attention has therefore tracked in great detail how health information systems (HIS) across the world have been established as a central tool for surveillance and modelling of disease trends, monitoring, and decision-making at the level of policy, planning, and resource allocation. This third and final section explores the production of health records in relation to State practices of regulating health. The authors go beyond descriptive studies of health information systems, and instead shed light on specific cultures of writing and knowledge production, as well as their performative effects on health and the construction of patient and care relations.

Senoo-Dogbey, Naab, and Akorfa Ohene open the section by providing detailed insights into the intersection of documentary and preventive practice in the context of professional care. Examining current evidence on Hepatitis B Virus (HBV) infection prevention practices among Health Care Workers (HCWs) in Ghana, the authors highlight the importance of documentation and the level of utilisation of data for decision-making under different components of the individual-level prevention practices. The chapter compares current practices regarding pre-exposure and post-exposure prophylaxis for HBV with recommended prevention practices outlined by the World Health Organization (WHO), the Centers for Disease Control and Prevention (CDC), as well as the Ghana Health Service (GHS). Doing so, the authors further examine the establishment of systems, structures, and programs at the health facility or hospital level to protect the health force from HBV infection. The chapter discusses gaps in practices at both the individual healthcare worker level and the facility level to protect healthcare workers from occupational exposures and subsequent infection with HBV. Narrowing in on prescriptive institutional preventive practices, Senoo-Dogbey, Naab, and Akorfa Ohene advance our understanding of how global best practices in recording risks and exposures are adapted in local settings, and bring about differential health outcomes in these contexts.

The final chapter in the volume explores Ghanaian health institutions' adoption and further development of digital platforms for the collection, aggregation, and analysis of health data. Thiel provides insights into the material and immaterial changes of an increasingly digital health sector, including its unintended consequences and recursive effects on professional knowledge practices. In so doing, the chapter sheds light on the bottom-up data practices that often invisibly (and in a taken-for-granted way) contribute to digital quantification. The chapter proceeds by narrowing in on the now well-established digital health information system DHIS2, and its role in the 2020 National Health Policy's goal of integrating determinants and institutions for holistic health outcomes. The evolution of digital health records in Ghana will be retraced, connecting a contemporary moment of transformation to the book's broader historical analyses. The chapter closes the book with a call for thick ethnographic observations of the (de)mobilising vectors and (de)synchronising effects of datafication, problematising its central promise of acceleration.

In sum, the contributions to this volume focus on routine health data and monitoring of diseases as they unfold in a historically variable and emerging health information infrastructure in Ghana. The book's interdisciplinary scope and design—combining perspectives from history, medical anthropology, sociology, and public health—discusses data practices ranging from the moment of diagnosis and codification of health-related information, record keeping, storage and retrieval for consultation, aggregation, reporting, decision-making, and health (policy) planning. Our investigations cover the (health) data practices of patients, clinical staff, ICT and health information systems experts, as well as regulators. Across this multiverse of registration and data practices, we explore the central role of knowledge infrastructures, as well as their navigations, adaptations, and deliberate mobilisations, as they have been historically folded into varying relations of coercion and autonomy. This, we hope, questions the contemporary hype around the datafication of health, demonstrating that it is neither new nor exceptional, but instead situated in a broader historical development of quantifying health in the interest of biopolitics.

References

AbouZahr, C., & Boerma, T. (2005). Health information systems: The foundations of public health. *Bulletin of the World Health Organization, 83*(7), 578–583.

Adam, V. (2016). *Metrics: What Counts in Global health*. Duke University Press.

Adu-Gyamfi, S., & Oware, R. (2019). Economy and health in the Gold Coast, 1902–1957. *African Economic History, 47*(2), 12–44.

Akyeampong, E. K., Hill, A. G., & Kleinman, A. (2015). *The culture of mental illness and psychiatric practice in Africa*. Indiana University Press.

Akyeampong, E. (2015). A historical overview of psychiatry in Africa. In E. Akyeampong, A. G. Hill, & A. Kleinman (Eds.), *The culture of mental illness and psychiatric practice in Africa* (pp. 24–49). Indiana University Press.

Al Dahdah, M., Desgrées Du Loû, A., & Méadel, C. (2015). Mobile health and maternal care: A winning combination for healthcare in the developing world? *Health Policy and Technology, 4*(3), 225–231.

Barry, A., & Born, G. (2014). *Interdisciplinarity: Reconfigurations of the social and natural sciences*. Routledge.

Behrends, A., Park, S.-J., & Rottenburg, R. (2014). *Travelling models in African conflict management: Translating technologies of social ordering*. Brill.

Beisel, U., Calkins, S., & Rottenburg, R. (2018). Divining, testing, and the problem of accountability. *HAU: Journal of Ethnographic Theory, 8*(1/2), 109–113.

Biruk, C. (2018). *Cooking data: Culture and politics in an African Research World*. Duke University Press.

Burchardt, M., & Umlauf, R. (2023). Where is the bottleneck? Drones and the paradoxes of digitising medical supplies in Ghana's landscapes of care. *Global Public Health, 18*(1), 2274434–2274434.

Csordas, T., & Lewton, E. (1998). Practice, performance, and experience in ritual healing. *Transcultural Psychiatry, 35*(4), 435–512.

Desrosières, A. (2015). Retroaction: How indicators feed back onto quantified actors. In R. Rottenburg, S. E. Merry, S.-J. Park, & J. Mugler (Eds.), *The world of indicators: The making of governmental knowledge through quantification. Cambridge studies in law and society* (pp. 329–353). Cambridge University Press.

Duclos, V. (2015). Global eHealth: Designing spaces of care in the era of global connectivity. *Medicine Anthropology Theory, 2*(1), 154–164.

Erikson, S. (2012). Global health business: The production and performativity of statistics in Sierra Leone and Germany. *Medical Anthropology, 31*(4), 367–384.

Feldman, K., Johnson, R. A., & Chawla, N. V. (2018). The state of data in healthcare: Path towards standardization. *Journal of Healthcare Informatics Research, 2*, 248–271.

Garfinkel, H. (2008). *Toward a sociological theory of information*. Paradigm Publishers.

Hoeyer, K., Bauer, S., Pickersgill, M., et al. (2019). Datafication and accountability in public health: Introduction to a special issue. *Social Studies of Science, 49*(4), 459–475.

Kehr, J., Dilger, H., & van Eeuwijk, P. (2018). Transfigurations of Health and the Moral Economy of Medicine: Subjectivities, Materialities, Values. *Zeitschrift Für Ethnologie, 143*(1), 1–20.

Kitchin, R. (2014). *The data revolution: A critical analysis of big data*. Sage.

Kleinman, A., & Benson, P. (2006). Anthropology in the clinic: The problem of cultural competency and how to fix it. *PLoS Medicine, 3*(10), Article e294. https://doi.org/10.1371/journal.pmed.0030294

Miscione, G., & Staring, K. (2009). Shifting ground for Health Information Systems: Local embeddedness, global fields, and legitimation. *International Journal of Sociotechnology and Knowledge Development, 1*(4), 1–12.

Ntewusu, S. (2020). *Corona in Ghana: A virus' impact on society and academic life*. African Studies Centre Leiden. Retrieved March 6, 2024, from https://www.ascleiden.nl/content/ascl-blogs/corona-ghana-virus-impact-society-and-academic-life

Patterson, A. (2018). *Africa and global health governance: Domestic politics and international structures*. Johns Hopkins University Press.

Prince, R. (2014). Situating health and the public in Africa: Historical and anthropological perspectives. In R. J. Prince & R. Marsland (Eds.), *Making and unmaking public health in Africa: Ethnographic perspectives* (pp. 1–54). Ohio University.

Rawls, A. W. (2008). Editor's introduction. In H. Garfinkel (Ed.), *Toward a sociological theory of information* (pp. 1–100). Paradigm Publishers.

Ruckenstein, M., & Dow Schüll, N. (2017). The datafication of health. *Annual Review of Anthropology, 46*(1), 261–278.

Ruppert, E., & Scheel, S. (2019). The politics of method: Taming the new, making data official. *International Political Sociology, 13*, 233–252.

Ruppert, E., & Scheel, S. (2021). *Data practices: making up a European people*. Goldsmiths Press.

Sæbø, J. I., Kossi, E. K., Titlestad, O. H., Tohouri, R. R., & Braa, J. (2011). Comparing strategies to integrate health information systems following a data warehouse approach in four countries. *Information Technology for Development, 17*(1), 42–60.

Siyam, A., Ir, P., York, D., Antwi, J., Amponsah, F., Rambique, O., Funzamo, C., Azeez, A., Mboera, L., Kumalija, C. J., & Rumisha, S. F. (2021). The burden of recording and reporting health data in primary health care facilities in five low- and lower-middle-income countries. *BMC Health Services Research, 21*(Suppl 1), 691. https://doi.org/10.1186/s12913-021-06652-5

Sund, R., Gissler, M., Hakulinen, T., & Rosén, M. (2014). Use of health registers. In W. Ahrens & I. Pigeot (Eds.), *Handbook of epidemiology* (pp. 707–730). Springer.

Thiel, A., & Agyekum, H. A. (2023). Crisis politics and the 2020 "Imposition of Restrictions Act" in Ghana. *Cahiers D'études Africaines, 250*, 363–383.

Warner, J. H. (1999). The uses of patient records by historians: Patterns, possibilities and perplexities. *Health and History, 1*(2/3), 101–102.

Whyte, S. R. (2011). Writing knowledge and acknowledgement: Possibilities in medical research. In W. Geissler (Ed.), *Evidence, ethos and experiment: The anthropology and history of medical research in Africa* (pp. 29–56). Berghahn Books.

Whyte, S. R. (2014). The publics of the new public health: Life conditions and "Lifestyle diseases" in Uganda. In R. J. Prince & R. Marsland (Eds.), *Making and unmaking public health in Africa: Ethnographic and historical perspectives* (pp. 187–207). Ohio University Press.

PART I

Health Data Histories

CHAPTER 2

Narratives on Health Policies in Northern Ghana: A note on British Colonial Policy and Local Knowledge Systems, 1902–1945

Oliver Kofi Tasin

2.1 Introduction

This chapter examines colonial health campaigns, and the role of ecology in discussions of health, in northern Ghana during the first half of the twentieth century. Northern Ghana in this study refers to the savanna ecological zone bordering Bono, Bono East, and Volta regions to the south, Ivory Coast to the west, Burkina Faso to the north, and Togo to the east. It therefore includes the contemporary Northern, Oti, Savanna, North East, Upper East, and Upper West regions. In the 1890s, northern Ghana referred to all areas to the north of Ashanti. In those days, the southern boundary ran roughly along the eighth parallel of latitude—though from 1906 the Black Volta River became the southern boundary to the west of Yeji (Watherston, 2008, p. 344). To the north and west of northern Ghana were the French territories of Upper Volta (Burkina

O. K. Tasin (✉)
St. Francis College of Education, Hohoe, Ghana
e-mail: oktasin@franco.edu.gh

A. Thiel and S. A. Ntewusu (eds.), *The Social Life of Health Data*,
https://doi.org/10.1007/978-981-97-3500-6_2

Faso) and Ivory Coast, respectively. To the east was German Togoland (later mandated to the British and French after 1918). In 1902, northern Ghana became part of three distinct but contiguous political units: the Gold Coast Colony (GCC) along the coastal areas, the Colony of Ashanti in the centre, and the Protectorate of the Northern Territories (a designation sometimes used interchangeably with northern Ghana) of the Gold Coast farther inland.[1]

Northern Ghana, therefore, lies wholly outside of the forest belt that stretches inland from the coast for about 200 miles, and is covered, in uncultivated parts, with rank grass. Its environmental conditions made northern Ghana prone to a host of diseases. The proximity of homes to rivers and streams made riverbanks breeding sites for disease vectors such as mosquitoes, tsetse flies, and blackflies. These prevailing environmental conditions increased the rate of diseases such as sleeping sickness, malaria, river blindness, and guinea worms. This chapter probes colonial health policies, particularly policies relating to sleeping sickness (i.e. trypanosomiasis, a disease transmitted by the tsetse fly), in northern Ghana from 1902 to 1945. It explores the processes through which colonial concepts of health captured indigenous knowledge of health conditions, diagnoses, and treatments. A host of actors, knowledge, and technologies of documenting health collaborated in measuring medical conditions in northern Ghana. This chapter focuses on the major shift in how health problems in northern Ghana and the colonial responses to them were conceptualised in the twentieth century. With this shift, the public health of African colonies became a global affair, as colonial health policies sought to tackle global health crises and epidemics across the territorial boundaries of States or colonies. As a result of the Northern Territories' interconnectedness with the external world, the public health of the indigenous population of northern Ghana and other African colonies became a matter of "global health" (Brown et al., 2006; Prince, 2013).

Using archival, oral history, and literature sources, this chapter chronicles a distinct path of health policies and inter-imperial studies in the first half of the twentieth century. The article contributes to a growing body of literature on colonial medical collaboration, and its application or relevance to inter-colonial studies and the response to diseases in Africa. It

[1] PRAAD (Accra) ADM 11/1/1160 Boundaries between the Gold Coast, Ashanti and the Northern Territories, 1912.

applies a transnational perspective to the various measures against diseases in the 1900s.

2.2 Indigenous Conceptualisation of Health

The World Health Organization (WHO) defines health as "the state of physical, mental and social wellbeing and not merely the absence of disease of infirmity" (Longley, 1996, p. 1, Adu-Gyamfi, 2013). Equally, medical anthropologists have distinguished between disease, sickness, and illness to foreground the social dynamics of health and healing. In that quest, "disease" stands for "organic pathologies and abnormalities," "illness" stands for "how diseases and sicknesses are brought into the individual's consciousness," and "sickness" stands for "the process through which worrisome behavioural, and biological signs, particularly ones originating from diseases are given socially recognized meanings" (Bortey Anum, 2015, p. 191). The definition of health as understood by clinical practitioners, however, tends to focus on physiological data, and devotes little attention to the social, performative, and ephemeral aspects of healing (Gemi-Iordanou, 2014, p. 1).

Clinical definitions of health influenced the way and manner in which health policies were developed and implemented by the British colonial administrators and medical practitioners in northern Ghana. In the meantime, the conception of health among the indigenous population of northern Ghana involves far more than the absence of disease and infirmities. For most ethnic groups in northern Ghana, apart from the general state of physical and social well-being, health also includes observance of religious and customary obligations, oaths to local chiefs, the maintenance of harmonious relations with family and social contacts, moderation in the consumption of certain types of food, and the acquisition of protective medicines.[2] It therefore integrates all dimensions of people's well-being, including how they interact with social institutions, ecology, and societal norms for healthy living (Tasin, 2018, p. 235, Russell, 1973). Health incorporates elements of personality and social skills, and reflects social

[2] Interview with Kumuncha Jagri, an 80-year-old Tigare healer, by Oliver Kofi Tasin on 5th June, 2022, at Kuwani in the Northern Region of Ghana.

norms and mutual support. For this reason, among the indigenous population of northern Ghana, to say a person does not possess wellness or health includes personal, familial, and societal conception of health.[3]

In this conceptualisation, the attainment of health is viewed as a relationship between social institutions, environmental practices, worldview, and the interrelation between the physical and the metaphysical aspects of a human being. It evokes complex relationships expressed and constructed by the indigenous population through performances in the maintenance of bodily health and well-being.[4] The performative aspect of healing includes the rites performed on individuals such as widows, widowers, orphans, and pregnant women to ensure their well-being. The inability of the society to achieve a social equilibrium through such social medication is regarded as ill-health or "dis-ease" suffered by a person or the society (Botchway, 2014, p. 161). Health and ill-health among the indigenous population of northern Ghana, therefore, went beyond a group of signs and symptoms inconsistent with normal order for a single person in a society, as construed by Western medicine. It was by this understanding and knowledge that various indigenous diseases were treated in indigenous contexts.

Not only did the indigenous population treat themselves; but earlier European travellers and missionaries were also treated and protected indigenously. For instance, Theophilus Opoku, a Basel missionary who contracted severe bouts of fever during his three-week stay in Salaga in 1877, was treated through indigenous methods (Gundona, 1999, p. 6). Similarly, Buss, a German visitor to Salaga who suffered from fever for a very long time in 1878, was cared for and treated by his landlord and other Muslims.[5] In 1888, when Curt Von Francois, another German colonial official, visited Salaga, he noted the prevalence of skin diseases and worms.[6] In the same way, George Ekem Ferguson reported the existence of dysentery, diarrhoea, colic, rheumatism, and guinea worm infection in the 1890s (Arhin, 1974, p. 80). Specifically regarding

[3] Interview with Beninbewir Gbenbor, 50 year old healer, by Oliver Kofi Tasin and Manee Maasund on 3rd January, 2017, at Nbuendo in the Savanes Region of Togo.

[4] Interview with Ugaja Bingnul, a 47-year-old healer, by Oliver Kofi Tasin on 23rd December, 2016, at Abunyanya in the Volta Region of Ghana.

[5] Marion Johnson, *Salaga Papers*, Vol. 1, No. SAL/9/2 (Legon: Institute of African Studies, University of Ghana).

[6] Johnson, *Salaga Papers*, Vol. 1, No. SAL/18/3.

smallpox, Curt Von Francois in 1888 reported its predominance and treatment among the indigenous population. He noted that:

> Among the infectious diseases, smallpox must be mentioned especially, which predominates for long periods. Several of the inhabitants have the reputations of being able to cure the sickness successfully.[7]

On the treatment of smallpox, he recounts:

> A brew of the leaves of a shrub is placed on the scabs. This reduces the suppuration. If they remain, the pocks are treated with an extract of the cooked root of the Gimon tree. Then the pocks dry up and are rubbed with shea butter. Healing follows after six weeks.[8]

Traditional rulers further enforced indigenous health and sanitation policies in northern Ghana such as communal labour, taboos, and other rules and regulations that helped to secure cleanliness and prevent diseases (Adu-Gyamfi et al., 2017, p. 2).

Despite the challenges of orality, health information among the indigenous population of northern Ghana was transmitted orally through time (Botchway, 2014, p. 170). They were not written down in medical treatises. It seems that this was so among many African societies. For example, this was true in the case of the Asante, whose medical culture, according to Botchway (2014, p. 170), "was not characterised by a corpus of ancient literary text and preserved manuscripts which contained written systems and theories that covered knowledge of life, health and disease of humans which were used by institutionally trained healers." Knowledge about the treatment of diseases was, as a result, acquired through daily observation and teaching, or through special training that was organised and executed by a practiced healer.

2.3 Colonial Health Regimes

Pioneering works by Scott (1965, 1983), Patterson (1981), Addae (1996a, 1996b), and Gale (1995) have traced the development of disease in Ghana during colonialism. Both Scott (1965) and Patterson (1981)

[7] Johnson, *Salaga Papers*, Vol. 1, No. SAL/18/3.

[8] Johnson, *Salaga Papers*, Vol. 1, No. SAL/18/3.

identify some of the socio-economic changes that influenced the battle against diseases on the Gold Coast during the first sixty years of the twentieth century. They link infectious diseases to human movement throughout history, and in particular note how explorers, merchants, soldiers, pilgrims, refugees, and migrants have carried plagues, measles, smallpox, typhoid, and a host of other deadly diseases across the globe. Their works stress that the besides the natural environment, mobility, urbanisation, and economic development have all had profound consequences for human health (Scott, 1965, p. 26). In line with this, S. K. Addae (1996a, 1996b) argues that the death rate of Europeans in the forts and castles across the coastal towns of Accra, Anomabo and Cape Coast prior to 1880 was excessively high. As a result, various European Merchant Companies sent surgeons to attend to the health needs of their countrymen in the Gold Coast. European missionary groups in the Gold Coast also used the quarantine method. From 1900 to 1960, Patterson (1981) observed the development of epidemiological methods in medical treatment. G. A. Ashitey (1994), Thomas S. Gale (1995), William H. Schneider (2009) and other colonial reports[9] note the colonial government's emphasis on vaccination as the main weapon of government efforts at disease control from the 1910s.

This shift was informed by considerable scientific research in colonial health at the beginning of the twentieth century, as well as political attention to the issue because of its importance to the conquest of sub-Saharan Africa by the European imperial powers. Most of these research missions started early in the preceding centuries, following the arrival of Europeans. The germ theory of disease began to predominate in many parts of the world (Tilley, 2016), and earlier breakthroughs of Louis Pasteur, Robert Koch, and Dmitri Ivanovsky in microbiology, bacteriology, and virology, respectively, in the late nineteenth century, further enhanced medical research in Africa (Botchway, 2014, p. 163; Smith, 2012, p. 5). Between 1901 and 1913, fifteen medical research missions (eight of them British) came to Africa to study various forms of diseases such as yaws, malaria, and sleeping sickness (Tilley, 2004).

These new ideas and techniques increased imperial powers' faith that diseases could be controlled and human lives prolonged, if only the

[9] N.A., "Health in Ghana," *The British Medical Journal*, Vol. 1, No. 5295 (1962); N.A., "Prevalence of Disease: Foreign Reports (1896–1970)," *Health Reports*, Vol. 59, No. 43, (1944).

new knowledge were utilised. By examining colonial health policies in northern Ghana, we can begin to understand the imperial machinations behind not only past interventions, but also contemporary health systems in African countries.

In northern Ghana, L. Wolf, a late nineteenth-century German explorer travelling through the Northern Territories observed that:

> Lack of water on the way was very noticeable; we drank avidly dirty water from puddles, which were to be found in shady bush holes. But I could not accustom myself to the little white worms or the little crab-like animals darting about as quick as lightening.[10]

According to him, these conditions were responsible for the prevalence of guinea worm that was so pronounced that he rarely met an African who did not show one or more symptoms of the worms. The best means to curb the prevalence of this disease was the provision of potable water. In his annual report, H. W. Leigh, Chief Commissioner of the Northern Territories (CCNT), recounted the provision of good and adequate water as one of the greatest and most urgent needs, which when supplied should do much to lessen guinea worm, ulcers, and various stomach diseases.[11] In a similar vein, a Director of Medical Services (DMS) in the Northern Territories stated:

> The outstanding need everywhere in the Northern Territories is an adequate supply of water of reasonably safe quality, whether the matter is considered from a preventive or a curative aspect or even from an economic aspect and apart from health. For a long time to come our chief efforts must be directed to coping with this need.[12]

[10] Johnson, *Salaga Papers*, Vol. 1, No. SAL/12/1.

[11] PRAAD (Tamale) NRG8/3/11 Annual Report on the Northern Territories of Gold Coast for the Year 1928–1929.

[12] PRAAD (Accra) CSO11/1/427 Medical and Sanitary Facilities in the Northern Territories, 1938.

2.4 The Case of Sleeping Sickness

Broadly, the climate and the diseases in West Africa made it uninhabitable to the early European explorers. The high level of European mortality in West Africa earned the region a Eurocentric title, "The White Man's Grave."[13] Doctor P.S. Selwyn-Clarke, the Gold Coast DMS, considered the Gold Coast Colony better in terms of trypanosomiasis concentration as compared to other colonies. He remarked: "I should like to make it clear that in my opinion trypanosomiasis on the Gold Coast is not so serious a matter as it is in Nigeria and elsewhere."[14] However, northern Ghana suffered more adverse effects from sleeping sickness than did the forest belt or the coast. The situation of sleeping sickness in northern Ghana was described as "hyperendemic" by the colonial administration.[15] By 1920s, district commissioners of northern Ghana began to report increasing numbers of infected people being brought to out-stations in search of medical assistance, and the corresponding mortalities.

The specific estimated figures as captured in the colonial records on the incidence of the disease in the Gold Coast from 1924 to 1934 are illustrated in Fig. 2.1.[16]

From Fig. 2.1, the prevalence of sleeping sickness only decreased in 1927–1928. All other years witnessed an increase in the level of the disease. By 1935, the stations with the greatest number of cases were Nankpandure (1012), Kumasi (252), Lawra (150), Bawku (96), Sunyani (96), Tamale (90), and Wa (77).[17] Sleeping sickness was, therefore, a public health problem of high magnitude in the British quest to establish colonies in Africa. Specifically, the spread of the disease among British

[13] PRAAAD (Accra) CSO11/1/371 Sanitation and Medical Facilities in the Gold Coast, 1934. For further information see, F. Harrison Rankin, The White Man's Grave: A Visit to Sierra Leone in 1834 (London: Richard Bentley, 1836), https://books.google.com, accessed 20 July 2022.

[14] PRAAD (Accra) CSO 11/19/04 Human Trypanosomiasis Reports on and measures to combat, 1934–1940.

[15] PRAAD (Accra) CSO 11/19/04 Human Trypanosomiasis Reports on and measures to combat, 1934–1940.

[16] PRAAD (Accra) CSO 11/19/04 Human Trypanosomiasis Reports on and measures to combat, 1934–1940.

[17] PRAAD (Accra) CSO 11/19/04 Human Trypanosomiasis Reports on and measures to combat, 1934–1940.

Year	Case	Deaths	Incidence per 10,000 of all cases treated
1924-25	26	—	3.2
1925-26	37	5	3.8
1926-27	67	11	6.4
1927-28	59	4	4.4
1928-29	94	18	5.3
1929-1930	121	23	6.6
1930-31	224	16	10.5
1931-32	250	28	12.6
1932-33	685	45	33.1
1933-34	1179	77	56.1

Fig. 2.1 Incidence of sleeping sickness distribution, 1924–1934

officials had reached such alarming proportion as to constitute a serious menace to the imperial ambition of the European powers.[18]

The years after 1935 saw an increase in the rate of the disease. In 1936, approximately 5,000 cases were confirmed in the Northern Territories, and village surveys suggested that infection rates were as high as 35–40% in some areas. The confirmed cases almost certainly represented a small fraction of the total number of people affected by the disease. Perhaps more importantly for prompting a reaction in Accra, several European officials were also infected, and the supply of migrant labourers to the Gold Coast's mines and cocoa plantations had begun to fall. Despite progressively energetic reactions from the 1930, delayed recognition of a sleeping sickness epidemic by the Gold Coast administration was partly due to a desire to preserve revenues and maintain the migrant labour supply to the south. Facing an undeniable epidemic, the government in Accra belatedly convened a committee on human trypanosomiasis. But it refused the proposed control measures of medical officers in northern Ghana, saying;

> The Committee, while agreeing that a large number of the labourers entering Ashanti from the Northern Territories are undoubtedly infected,

[18] PRAAD (Accra) CSO 11/19/14 The Incidence and Distribution of Human Trypanosomiasis in British Tropical Africa, 1939.

> is unable to envisage any system of regulation which might be expected to succeed ... any such scheme of control might interfere with the free flow of labour towards the mines, which are likely to make increasingly heavy demands upon the NTs as a source of supply.[19]

Thus official recognition of any epidemic disease could entail a substantial loss of income, when it mandated the imposition of quarantine and control measures under local or international law. For instance, under the International Sanitary Conventions of 1912 and 1926, confirmation of a small set of "notifiable diseases" meant that a country, port or city declared as "infected" could be subject to the suspension of trade.[20] The conventions did not include sleeping sickness, nor many other infectious diseases prevalent in Africa. But international notification of any epidemic could still act as a general deterrent to commerce, and neighbouring countries might be compelled to prevent their subjects from entering an "infected" region.[21]

Consequently, the British efforts to create export economies had adverse effects on the health of the indigenous population of northern Ghana. In line with the capitalist colonial ideology, locals were enlisted into mining, infrastructure, and agricultural projects with few occupational protections and succumbed to illnesses that resulted from their labour.[22] Additionally, workers experienced diseases such as tuberculosis in the mining towns of the south. In areas of large-scale shea tree and other agricultural plantations, the local population became more vulnerable to water-borne, mosquito-borne, and worm-borne diseases emerging from the altered environments.[23] Even though the Northern Territories Rivers Ordinance (NTRO), passed in 1903, was supposed to regulate activities on the water bodies in the Northern Territories, the ordinance did not fully achieve its aim. In particular, the ordinance gave license and empowered the colonial government to dredge for minerals and precious

[19] PRAAD (Accra) CSO 11/19/14 The Incidence and Distribution of Human Trypanosomiasis in British Tropical Africa, 1939.

[20] PRAAD (Accra), CSO11/10/8 Records of Infectious Diseases, 1931–1932.

[21] PRAAD (Accra), CSO11/10/8 Records of Infectious Diseases; 1931–1932; PRAAD (Accra), CSO11/10/9 Records of Infectious Diseases, 1932–1934.

[22] PRAAD (Tamale) NRG8/3/103 Annual Report for Northern Territories, 1940–1941.

[23] PRAAD (Tamale) NRG8/3/49 Annual Report for Northern Territories, 1934–1935.

stones in the Northern Territories.[24] Subsequently, in 1904, the Mineral Rights Ordinance (MRO) was passed. This ordinance further gave colonial government the right to engage in mining activities in northern Ghana. The ordinance specifically states:

> The area for which an application for a mining option is made shall be defined by true bearings or by well marked natural or artificial features which can be identified both on the ground and in a published map, and in all cases must start from some easily defined point, which may be either a natural feature such as a prominent rock, or else a cairn or pillar erected by the applicant for the option. The Chief Commissioner shall on receipt of any such application by the holder of a prospecting option issue to the applicant as many mining options in the prescribed form as the applicant requires over as many blocks of land not exceeding five square miles each, as have been defined in the application, subject to the prescribed conditions and to any conditions with regard to dealings with native chiefs or any native person he may think fit to impose.[25]

Mining and other colonial activities produced outcomes in contrast with the goals of the British campaign against diseases in northern Ghana. As demand for industrial labourers increased, it equally led to significant urban drift from northern Ghana, with its corollary effects.[26] Colonial exploitation of mineral and agricultural resources there contributed to the emergence of some diseases. In the case of sleeping sickness, however, it was concentrated in northern Ghana. For example, a report on sleeping sickness for 1933–1934 showed a ratio of 7.1 per ten thousand patients treated in the coastal zone. In the forest belt the ratio showed an increase to 84.7 per ten thousand patients treated, whilst the incidence in the savannah belt was at a ratio of 87.3 per ten thousand.[27] This shows a progressive increase in the prevalence of the disease as one moves towards the Sahelian region.

[24] PRAAD (Accra) ADM 4/1/32 Ordinances of Northern Territories, 1903.

[25] PRAAD (Accra) ADM 4/1/33 Ordinances of the Gold Coast Ashanti and Northern Territories, 1904.

[26] PRAAD (Accra) CSO 21/4/46 Visit of Northern Territories Chiefs to the Mines in the Colony, 1940.

[27] PRAAD (Accra) CSO 11/19/04 Human Trypanosomiasis Reports on and measures to combat, 1934–1940.

Unlike venereal diseases, which were transported from the south to the north through labour returnees, cases of sleeping sickness were transported from the north to the south. In the view of Doctor P.S. Selwyn-Clarke, DMS, "there is some evidence to suggest that in both coastal and forest cases a certain proportion of the sufferers are immigrants from endemic or epidemic areas in the Northern Territories of the Gold Coast or from neighbouring French territory."[28] Northern Ghana and neighbouring regions were largely responsible for the bulk of the cases in southern towns such as Sunyani, Kitampo, and Kumasi.

2.5 Colonial Responses to Sleeping Sickness in Northern Ghana

Apart from Kumasi and Sunyani, the urban centres of epidemics of sleeping sickness were located in northern Ghana. The coastal towns such as Cape Coast, Accra, and Sekondi-Takoradi had minimal incidence of sleeping sickness. Remarking on the challenging nature of the health situation in the Northern Territories, the Chief Commissioner of the Northern Territories (CCNT) said the fact that disease is a serious menace to the future welfare of the protectorate was beyond question, and that steps must be taken for its suppression and eventual eradication.[29] The disease was taken as an administrative question of major importance to the British colonial administration. In the opinion of G. Saunders and K. S. Morris, colonial entomologists in northern Ghana, diseases such as "trypanosomiasis constitutes a continual drain and ill-health; and also that there is a potential danger of extension."[30] In their view, if the development of the country were to progress, then measures must be adopted in such a way as not to expose large number of people to various infectious diseases and vectors of such diseases. It was in pursuit of such general goals that the British responded through therapeutic and preventive measures.

[28] PRAAD (Accra) CSO 11/19/04 Human Trypanosomiasis Reports on and measures to combat, 1934–1940.

[29] PRAAD (Accra) CSO 11/19/04 Human Trypanosomiasis Reports on and measures to combat, 1934–1940.

[30] PRAAD (Accra) CSO11/19/2 Tsetse Fly investigation in the Gold Coast, 1930–1932.

Colonial administrators were aware of indigenous diagnoses carried out before the indigenous population sought western medical care. H. C. Armstrong, the Medical Officer of Health (MOH), in his annual address described sleeping sickness and malaria as "home diseases" in northern Ghana, such that it was the duty of the individual to kill tsetse flies and mosquitoes.[31] Batchelor, a colonial official in the 1930s, confirmed indigenous knowledge of sleeping sickness and its diagnosis in his report on the method of diagnosis. He recounts:

> It should be realised that practically every patient came to hospital with a self-made diagnosis of trypanosomiasis and the diagnosis was almost always confirmed. These people now have a good knowledge of this disease as natives elsewhere have of yaws.[32]

Nonetheless, the approach by the colonial government first emphasised the diagnosis of diseases and their causes among the indigenous population. The diagnosis of human African trypanosomiasis, in the colonial response, required a high degree of training and expertise. Initially, the parasite must be detected. This relied on conventional techniques such as lymph node puncture, blood film examination, or various elaborate techniques (Stich et al., 2002, p. 204). Patients were given the standard form of treatment, three one-gramme doses of antrypol or Bayer 205 followed by five two-gramme doses of tryparsamide. For instance, in 1933, an estimated number of 1,186 patients were treated, with 741 being inpatients and 445 being outpatients, and 1,973 were treated in 1934, with 1,449 being inpatients and 524 outpatients.[33]

The preventive approach was regarded as the most important part of any work against malaria, trypanosomiasis, and other diseases. This principally entailed a focus on the promotion of good sanitation and hygiene. This called for the implementation of the policy of clearing by the colonial administration. In a note from the Director of Medical Services' visit to the Northern Territories, he reports;

[31] ARG1/19/6 Minutes of the Annual Conference of Officers in the Northern Territories held at Tamale, 1921–1924, December 1937.

[32] PRAAD (Accra) CSO 11/19/11 Inoculation of certain People at Bawku for Sleeping Sickness, 1937.

[33] PRAAD (Accra) CSO 11/19/04 Human Trypanosomiasis Reports on and measures to combat, 1934–1940.

> Dr. K. Morris has evolved a method of eradication of fly belt by means described as 'selective clearing of vegetation.' This, in fact, amounts in principle to the partial clearing of such belts by the removal only of such trees and other vegetation, as his experience and study have led him to regard, as the sole factors in maintaining the localised climates necessary to the continued existence of the two principal vectors of human trypanosomiasis in the Colony, namely Glossina palpalis and Glossina tachinoides.[34]

In a letter from the Colonial Secretary to the Chief Commissioner of the Northern Territories (CCNT) dated 8th June 1944, the CCNT was to adopt Morris' method of Kamba clearing and settlement scheme, which included the settlement of men and families on the rehabilitated areas. Some of the military men who returned from the World War II were also resettled in some of these rehabilitated areas.[35] It was not regarded as efficient or the most beneficial method to rely upon treatment alone to eradicate the disease; hence, controlled clearing was of paramount importance. It became the duty of the colonial entomologist who investigated the extent to which clearing was done, and with trained staff, supervised the communal labour.[36] The clearing was initially extended 50 yards around a water hole, and 100 yards on either side of a main road crossing a stream. Batchelor further recommended the extension to be increased to 100 yards around a water hole and 150 yards on either side of main roads crossing streams and rivers.[37]

Yet colonial health practices did not always produce the intended outcomes. As Bannister (2021) shows, the colonial quest to control sleeping sickness uncontrollably led to the emergence of an eye disease known as river blindness, or onchocerciasis. This was due to the fact that the colonial government in the Northern Territories invariably focused on the sleeping sickness treatment campaign, which unexpectedly obscured the extent of onchocerciasis infection (Bannister, 2021, p. 56).

[34] PRAAD (Accra) CSO 11/16/76 Trypanosomiasis, 1944–1945.

[35] PRAAD (Accra) CSO 11/16/76 Trypanosomiasis, 1944–1945.

[36] PRAAD (Tamale) NRG8/13/16 Tsetse Control, 1950–1955.

[37] PRAAD (Accra) CSO 11/19/11 Inoculation of certain People at Bawku for Sleeping Sickness, 1937.

2.6 Health and Colonial Cooperation

The nature of health conditions led to the need for intra-colonial and inter-colonial cooperation between the British colonial government and other authorities. While the motives of European powers differed, they tended to be optimistic about the potential wealth of the new territories in terms of both natural resources and labour pools (Tilley, 2016, p. 744). Campaign against diseases took on an important role given the mandate of "improving" the health conditions of Africans (Tilley, 2016, p. 744). However, the European effort to decrease the health challenges through campaigns was faced with multiple difficulties. It necessitated massive coordinated efforts by imperial powers within disease-endemic territories to form cooperation among other European powers such as the British, French, Germans, and Belgians, non-governmental organisations, and other agencies in order to improve health conditions, and such cooperation included the indigenous authorities, in line with the indirect rule policy.[38] As argued by the DMS in 1934, the epidemic that required the closest cooperation between the government and other authorities was trypanosomiasis.[39]

Where there were challenges in examining people, the chiefs were to convince their subjects to make themselves available for examination. As emphasised by Kelburne K. Grieve, DDMS, the cooperation of the political officers was an absolute necessity, and the British needed the assistance of the chiefs in order to implement various health campaigns.[40] Similarly, the DMS observed;

> I think that if we can get various Native Authorities to look after themselves, i.e. their own riverine clearings, fords, water-holes, etc., it will be as much as we shall ever get out of them. I do not consider that they will ever

[38] Indirect rule was a British administrative system whereby local administration was entrusted to indigenous people and institutions with the supervision and an overriding authority of the governor (see Apter 1955, p. 123).

[39] PRAAD (Accra) CSO 11/19/04 Human Trypanosomiasis Reports on and measures to combat, 1934–1940.

[40] PRAAD (Accra) CSO 11/19/04 Human Trypanosomiasis Reports on and measures to combat, 1934–1940.

efficiently make and maintain clearings on the main trade routes, possibly far removed from their own immediate environment.[41]

The cooperation also manifested in the series of international health conferences that were held at the beginning of the twentieth century. For instance, at the first International Conference on Sleeping Sickness (ICSS) in 1907, Lord Fitz-Maurice, the president of the conference, emphasised concerted cooperation among the imperial powers. In his remarks at the opening of the meeting to describe the object in view, he stated, "we are meeting together in the hope that it may be possible to concert measures which will enable the Powers which we represent to wage a more effective warfare against that terrible epidemic of sleeping sickness, which has already devastated so great a part of Africa, and which appears to be assuming even greater and greater proportions."[42] The main aim of such conferences was to curb epidemics and diseases in the first half of the twentieth century.

The existence of several important loci of epidemics and the mobility of such epidemics in British, German, and French territories made cooperation cardinal. Inter-colonial cooperation was aimed at dealing with reinvasion from neighbouring territories. J. L. W. Fynn argued that, "even if one country were to clean up its own tsetse areas, it would still be subject to the danger of re-invasion from outside, unless her neighbours took similar steps at the same time."[43] This made inter-colonial cooperation essential in the quest to completely eradicate tsetse flies across neighbouring colonies. In the case of northern Ghana, the British cooperated and signed agreements with the French and the Germans. In 1911, the British and German governments signed an agreement to cooperate on sleeping sickness measures on both sides of their frontiers. The agreement was undoubtedly a happy gesture, but it was not of great practical value and lapsed with the outbreak of the First World War.[44] The aim

[41] PRAAD (Accra) CSO 11/19/04 Human Trypanosomiasis Reports on and measures to combat, 1934–1940.

[42] *Nature*, June 20, 1907, p. 188, https://www.nature.com/articles/076188a0.pdf, accessed 2 July 2022.

[43] PRAAD (Accra) CSO 11/19/04 Human Trypanosomiasis Reports on and measures to combat, 1934–1940.

[44] PRAAD (Accra) CSO 11/19/04 Human Trypanosomiasis Reports on and measures to combat, 1934–1940.

of the agreement was to combat sleeping sickness in the Gold Coast Colony, the Ashanti Protectorate, the Northern Territories of the Gold Coast, and in Togoland. The agreement provided for new investigations of the disease and intensified programmes of treatment, closure of borders and trade, and restrictions on the movement of African peoples between the two colonies (Eckart, 2002). Along with the quarantine measures described above, the agreement itself suggests that sleeping sickness in the early twentieth-century Gold Coast had a greater impact than has earlier been recognised.

The focus of the German Imperial Government was in the neighbourhood of Misahoe and the area that stretched as far as Sansane Mango, a town in Togoland not far from the border of British northern Ghana. It was in the quest to prevent cross-border mobility of diseases that the French established a series of camps. It is worth noting that the Germans had established a sleeping sickness camp in Togoland in 1903 (Eckart, 2002, p. 79). In 1908, a second camp was formed on the Kluto plateau in Togoland, and some 593 cases were dealt with there up to 1913. Von Raven, a German colonial official, described the inmates of the Kluto camp as not being "disciplined" and "willing" as he had hoped for (Eckart, 2002, p. 85). News of indiscipline in the camps, in particular, were to be blamed for the challenges in handling sleeping sickness in German territories. The situation, where news was spread by patients who had been sent back home for "observation," made the management of patients in the camps difficult. As a result, the disease, both inside and outside the camps, threatened the total population (Eckart, 2002, p. 85).

It was due to such collaboration that the League of Nations Health Organization (LNHO) Expert Committee on sleeping sickness was established in 1922. This was followed by an International Conference on Sleeping Sickness, held in London in 1925 under the auspices of the League, that shared ideas on how to tackle the ravages of the disease (Coghe, 2014, p. 139). Such conferences further promoted inter-imperial studies on sleeping sickness by doctors of the imperial powers from the 1930s.

2.7 Colonial Health Documentation

Of central importance to inter-colonial studies of health was the need for statistical records and records keeping. In a report by the Committee on Human Trypanosomiasis issued in 1935, the committee lamented the lack of authoritative data on the subject of trypanosomiasis in the Gold Coast. It further states, "it is important that the whole territory should be made the subject of a special survey so as to provide statistics which should form the basis of comparison with data obtained in subsequent years."[45] G. F. T. Saunders, in his visit to Dakar in 1936, suggested the method of dual registration that entailed registration with the medical officials and with the chief of an area. In his view, registration of cases with both the imperial power and the chief of the area was essential. Saunders' policy in the case of the Gold Coast was to refuse infected patients from French territory, unless personally known to a chief in British territory.[46] This meant that close village-to-village work was key in keeping health records of contagious or infective endemic disease. In some cases, voluntary workers played a partial role in keeping records. As indicated in Saunders' report,

> Every patient is fully examined by a pupil or volunteer worker and detailed notes taken. The doctor then goes over these notes with a group of two or three pupils and discussion is allowed. The form on which the notes are written is a large one, with a vertical line marking off a space for treatment. The treatment ordered is then written in the space provided, side by side with the examination. Each day observation made and treatment prescribed are noted in the same way.[47]

The Medical Officer had, of course, the salutary exercise of writing his case in the "case book" as a means of keeping health information. This was complemented by records the chiefs kept of who they had required to swear an oath; this oath was intended to prevent patients from absconding, and to keep them at treatment camps until they were treated fully. G. L. Alexander, Medical Officer in the northern Ghana, succinctly captured such behaviour:

> Last year a high proportion absconded as soon as they felt better after a few injections. We are now having very little trouble with them in this way. At Bawku, the practice is to take new patients to the chief, and make them give him an undertaking that they will remain until discharged. Then if

[45] PRAAD (Accra) CSO 11/16/76 Trypanosomiasis, 1944–1945.

[46] PRAAD (Accra) CSO 11/19/04 Human Trypanosomiasis Reports on and measures to combat, 1934–1940.

[47] PRAAD (Accra) CSO 11/19/04 Human Trypanosomiasis Reports on and measures to combat, 1934–1940.

> they do abscond, the chief is asked to have them brought back. At Nakpanduri, a native administration police officer has been stationed, whose duty it is to go after defaulters.[48]

The cooperation between colonial administration and the indigenous authorities was key in administering treatments. It is worth noting that many of the patients at the treatment camps such as Nakpanduri came from a long distance. This made it difficult for them to maintain their food supplies. Since they were not fed due to the cost of feeding all the patients, some obviously resorted to absconding the moment they felt better. Another challenge encountered by the colonial regime was the designation of the disease as a reproach and disgrace among some of the indigenous population.[49] This meant that individuals suspected of being infected with sleeping sickness neither went to the hospital nor allowed themselves to be examined. As a result, latent cases could not be discovered early.

Despite the fact that the indigenous people of northern Ghana had no written texts of their own on public health policies, they maintained their health practices through oaths. These oaths, to borrow the words of Murray Last (1999, p. 75), were not the invention of biomedicine but of the primary outlook of an indigenous medical system. They were taken under the controlling power of public healers who addressed a series of health problems such as epidemics, fertility, famine, and the promotion of sanitation practices as well as health education. The commitment of the indigenous population not to break such oaths promoted their adherence to such public health policies. Such policies were emic in nature, in other words from an insider's perspective (Warren, 1975, p. 117), and consisted of a culture-specific ideology of health and health behaviours.

2.8 Conclusion

Due to environmental conditions, the indigenous population of northern Ghana has long been faced with the challenge of fighting against diseases. Indigenous approaches to the treatment of diseases were rooted in

[48] PRAAD (Accra) CSO 11/19/04 Human Trypanosomiasis Reports on and measures to combat, 1934–1940.

[49] PRAAD (Accra) CSO 11/19/11 Inoculation of certain People at Bawku for Sleeping Sickness, 1937.

their cosmology, and the desire to eradicate such diseases was aimed at promoting societal well-being in order to ensure the continuity of the society. The British quest to extend health care and eradicate common diseases differed radically from this conceptualisation of health, but British policy also differed between northern Ghana and other parts of Ghana. Initially ignored in terms of the provision of health care, northern Ghana experienced a change in policy by the British after the First World War, due to the desire for stable human resource flows. A stable population that could support the British in defence and also serve as a reservoir for the supply of labour became paramount to colonial health policy. In that regard, the colonial medical approach and the quest to prevent disease in the twentieth century was built on achieving the socio-economic aims of the British and other imperial powers. Initially limited to only the Europeans, promotion of health was thus gradually extended to the African population, in the quest for British imperial success.

Although some earlier researchers have examined the concept of health in northern Ghana, the broader implications of transnational collaboration and inter-imperial learning call for further enquiry. The colonial failure to incorporate local knowledge of diseases into its wide net of collaborations strongly symbolises colonial prejudice regarding indigenous medical knowledge. Control over healing was central to the social and political power exercised by either a healer or traditional leader. In this regard, indigenous healers also served as a check on the powers of political leaders. However, colonial suppression of indigenous medical practices, and the exile of some indigenous healers and leaders, destroyed such forms of knowledge. In line with Prince et al. (2013, p. 16), the colonial regime reduced all aspects of African medical knowledge to that of timeless, archaic tradition, and sought to render healers' practices illegal. Such measures of repression reflected the presumptions of colonial medical imperialism in Africa. The vehicles for these ideas and experiments were seen in the nature of health policies and ordinances passed by the regime throughout the colonial period, and were cemented in routine statistical and reporting practice. They illustrate graphically how the various means of curbing diseases as employed by the British were not humane in their goals, but aimed at attaining the central imperial ambitions of the British.

Conflict of Interest No conflict of interest is declared.

References

Primary Sources

Oral Interviews

Bingnul, Ugaja. 47 year old healer, interviewed by Oliver Kofi Tasin on 23rd December, 2016, at Abunyanya in the Volta Region of Ghana.

Gbenbor, Beninbewir. 50 year old healer, interviewed by Oliver Kofi Tasin and Manee Maasund on 3rd January, 2017, at Nbuendo in the Savanes Region of Togo.

Jagri, Kumuncha. 80 year old healer through *Tigari*, interviewed by Oliver Kofi Tasin on 5th June, 2022, at Kuwani in the Northern Region of Ghana.

Archival Sources

PRAAD, Accra

PRAAD (Accra) ADM 4/1/33 Ordinances of the Gold Coast Ashanti and Northern Territories, 1904

PRAAD (Accra) ADM 4/1/40 Ordinances of the Gold Coast Ashanti and Northern Territories, 1911

ADM 11/1/1160 Boundaries between the Gold Coast, Ashanti and the Northern Territories

ADM 56/1/52 Northern Territories Administration.

CSO11/1/371 Sanitation and Medical Facilities in the Gold Coast

CSO 11/16/76 Trypanosomiasis

CSO 11/19/02 Tsetse Fly Investigation in the Gold Coast

CSO 11/19/07 Anti-tsetse fly work

CSO 11/19/04 Human Trypanosomiasis Reports on and measures to combat

CSO 11/19/9 Anti-trypanosomiasis campaigns

CSO 11/19/11 Inoculation of certain People at Bawku for Sleeping Sickness

CSO 11/19/12 Anti-trypanosomiasis injections

CSO 11/19/14 The Incidence and Distribution of Human Trypanosomiasis in British Tropical Africa.

PRAAD (Accra) CSO 21/4/46 Visit of Northern Territories Chiefs to the Mines in the Colony, 1940

PRAAD, Cape Coast

ADM23/1/368 Provincial Board of Health.

ADM23/1/2192 Central Health Board

PRAAD, Kumasi

ARG1/19/6 Minutes of the Annual Conference of Officers in the Northern Territories held at Tamale, 21–24 December 1937.

PRAAD, Tamale

NRG2/20/1 Tsetse fly Clearing
PRAAD (Tamale) NRG8/3/49 Annual Report for Northern Territories, 1934–1935
PRAAD (Tamale) NRG8/3/103 Annual Report for Northern Territories, 1940–1941
NRG8/13/9 Rural Medical Services
NRG8/13/16 Tsetse Control
NRG8/13/34 Northern Territories Health Board.

Secondary Sources

Addae, S. (1996a). *The evolution of modern medicine in a developing country: Ghana, 1880–1960*. Durham Academic Press.

Addae, S. (1996b). *History of western medicine in Ghana, 1880–1960*. Durham Academic Press.

Adu-Gyamfi, S. (2013). A historical review of disease prevention in Gold Coast: Focus on Asante (1900–1957). *Historical Research Letter, 5*, 1–39.

Adu-Gyamfi, S., Brenya, E., & Egyir, P. N. (2017). Public health in colonial and post-colonial Ghana: Lesson-drawing for the twenty-first century. *Studies in Arts and Humanities, 3*(1), 1–21.

Apter, D. E. (1955). *The Gold Coast in transition*. Princeton University Press.

Arhin, K. (1974). The papers of George Ekem Ferguson, A Fanti Official of the Government of the Gold Coast, 1890–1897. *African Social Research Documents*, 7. Afrika-Studiecentrum Leiden.

Ashitey, G. A. (1994). *Disease control in Ghana: An epidemiology of disease control in Ghana 1901–1990*. Ghana Universities Press.

Bannister, D. (2021). The Sorcerer's apprentice: Sleeping sickness, onchocerciasis, and unintended consequences in Ghana. *Journal of African History, 62*(1), 29–57.

Bortey, A. E. N. (2015). The Placebo phenomenon and the Jesus factor in healing practices in Ghana. In J. B. A. Afful, Grant, P., de-Souza, A., & Gborsong, P. A. (Eds.), *Communication, culture and health* (pp. 185–196). University of Cape Coast Press.

Botchway, D. N. Y. M. (2014). A note on the ethnomedical universe of the Asante, an indigenous people in Ghana. In E. Gemi-Iordanou, Gordon, S.,

Matthew, R., McInnes, E., & Pettitt, R. (Eds.), *Healing and performance* (pp. 160–175). Oxbow Books.

Brown, T. M., Cueto, M., & Fee, E. (2006). The World Health Organization and the transition from "International" to "Global" Public Health. *American Journal of Public Health, 96*(1), 62–72.

Coghe, S. (2014). Inter-imperial learning and African Health Care in Portuguese Angola in the Interwar Period. *Social History of Medicine, 28*(1), 134–154.

Eckart, W. U. (2002). The colony as laboratory: German sleeping sickness campaigns in German East Africa and in Togo, 1900–1914. *History and Philosophy of the Life Sciences, 24*(1), 69–89.

Gale, T. S. (1995). The struggle against disease in the Gold Coast: Early attempts at urban sanitary reform. *Transactions of the Historical Society of Ghana, 16*(2), 185–203.

Gemi-Iordanou, E., Gordon, S., Matthew, R., McInnes, E., & Pettitt, R. (2014). *Medicine*. Oxbow Books.

Gundona, S. (1999). A study of health conditions and disease control in the Northern Territories of the Gold Coast, 1897–1956. MPhil Thesis, University of Ghana, Legon.

Last, M. (1999). Understanding health. In T. Allen & T. Skelton (Eds.), *Culture and global change* (pp. 70–84). Routledge.

Longley, D. (1996). *Health care constitutions*. Cavendish Publishing Ltd.

Patterson, D. K. (1981). *Health in colonial Ghana: Disease, medicine and socio-economic change, 1900–1955*. Crossroads Press.

Prince, R. J. (2013). Situating health and the publics in Africa: Historical and anthropological perspectives. In R. J. Prince & R. Marsland (Eds.), *Making and unmaking public health in Africa: Ethnographic and historical perspectives* (pp. 1–51). Ohio University Press.

Russell, R. D. (1973). Social health: An attempt to clarify this dimension of well-being. *International Journal of Health Education, 16*, 74–82.

Schneider, W. H. (2009). Smallpox in Africa during colonial rule. *Medical History, 53*, 193–227.

Scott, D. (1965). *Epidemic disease in Ghana, 1901–1960*. Oxford University Press.

Scott, D. (1983). The influenza epidemic of 1918–19 in the Gold Coast. *The Journal of African History, 24*(4), 485–502.

Smith, K. A. (2012). Louis Pasteur, the Father of Immunology? *Frontiers in Immunology, 3*(69), 1–10.

Stich, A., Abel, P. M., & Krishna, S. (2002). Human African Trypanosomiasis. *BMJ: British Medical Journal, 325*(7357), 203–206.

Tasin, O. K. (2018). Change and continuity of Konkomba medical culture: A historical perspective of an Indigenous People in Northern Ghana. *Abibisem: Jounal of African Culture and Civilization, 7*, 211–248.

Tilley, H. (2004). Ecologies of complexity: Tropical environments, African Trypanosomiasis, and the science of disease control in British Colonial Africa, 1900–1940. *Osiris, 19*, 21–38.

Tilley, H. (2016). Medicine, empires, and ethics in colonial Africa. *AMA Journal of Ethics, 18*(7), 743–753.

Warren, D. M. (1975). The role of emic analyses in medical anthropology: The case of the Bono of Ghana. *Anthropological Linguistics, 17*(3), 117–126.

Watherston, A. E. G. (2008). The Northern territories of the Gold Coast. *Journal of the Royal African Society, 7*(28), 344–373.

CHAPTER 3

"Campaign": A History of the Medial Field Unit in Ghana

Samuel Aniegye Ntewusu

3.1 Introduction

In colonial times, a Medical Field Unit (MFU) was a broad categorisation referring to a group of health workers who provided basic health services. One could liken the MFU to a mobile health unit with some form of medical care, in which the services were brought to the patient rather than having the patient travel to the services (Bodenheimer, 1969, p. 144). The MFU could be as simple as a medically-trained person bringing his or her talent to the patient's home, or as complex as a fully-equipped medical team with multiple personnel.

D. Scott, a specialist epidemiologist for the Medical Field Unit in Ghana, identified two characteristics of the Medical Field Units in different historical periods. According to him, initially the MFUs were not termed as such, but rather were simply regarded as mobile field units responsible for providing dispensary services in remote areas. Sometimes this involved one person being in charge of an entire district

S. A. Ntewusu (✉)
University of Ghana, Accra, Ghana
e-mail: santewusu@ug.edu.gh

A. Thiel and S. A. Ntewusu (eds.), *The Social Life of Health Data*,
https://doi.org/10.1007/978-981-97-3500-6_3

comprising about ten thousand inhabitants. Examples include the posting of Mr. Musa Kalinsi, an ex-serviceman, to the Nawuri area in Kpandai, East Gonja District of the present-day Northern Region. His duties included dressing sores in the case of leprosy, and antenatal services. The second phase, which Scott regarded as the MFU's real flowering, was the response to the human trypanosomiasis (sleeping sickness) epidemic over the whole of West Africa in the 1930s and 1940s (Scott, 1962, p. 19). It therefore was a West African concept which was developed simultaneously in many different countries in the region in response to a common danger. Nonetheless, Mengistu Misganaw (2006, p. 35) points out that Medical Field Units were population-specific, and well-focused in terms of definition and practice. Their operation adopted a holistic approach in considering the broad range of interacting needs that affect the collective health of the client, where the client is a composite of people whose relationships and interactions with each other must be considered in totality.

This chapter adds to these perspectives and insights by discussing the history of the Medical Field Units in the Gold Coast, and their contribution to the capture of medical knowledge. The chapter presents an analysis of their categories of staff, their areas of operation, their focal diseases, and their operational problems. The intent is to provide perspectives on the general survey of the field of endemic disease through different categories of staff, fields of specialisation, administrative duties, and areas of operation. It will be shown how data generation was crucial to the functioning of the MFU. Such data generated relevant sources for historical discussion. But it also provides an avenue into the analysis of colonial health services, their organisation of expertise, the infrastructure mobilised to produce certain knowledges in the fight against diseases in the different regions of Ghana, and the substantial infrastructural and logistical problems involved in the operations of health systems such as the MFU.

Methodologically, this chapter relies on archival sources and interviews as well as published material to construct the history of Medical Field Units in Ghana. Among Ghana's several archives, the Public Records and Archives Administration (PRAAD), both in their wide range of topics and their accessibility, are an invaluable tool for Ghana's social and economic history. Currently, PRAAD has eight different branches countrywide, including the National Archive in Accra, which doubles as the Greater Accra regional archive. There is one archive in each region, with the exception of the Upper East and the Upper West regions. The documents for the Upper regions were accommodated in Tamale. This is not surprising since these two regions were carved out of the Northern Region. The newer region, the Upper West, was created in 1988 (Ntewusu, 2014). In dealing with the MFU, I visited the Accra and Tamale offices of PRAAD. The use of the archives in this chapter is informed by an academic tradition in historiographical studies which consists of several general principles, including searching for materials that modify hypotheses with a verification, and representing evidence as it is contained in the archives. The archival material presented here provides basic information related to the MFU. It enabled the production of a historiographical picture of the operation of the MFU, as well as their social context. The graphs produced throughout this chapter provide an exhibition of the history of the MFU in Ghana.

As stated, the Medical Field Units in Ghana were formally known as the Trypanosomiasis Campaign. The Campaign started in the mid-1930s, following the outbreak of sleeping sickness in most parts of northern Ghana. In 1951, B.B. Waddy was put in charge of the Trypanosomiasis Campaign of the Gold Coast. He was tasked by the then Director of Medical Services, Dr R.L Cheverton, to change its name to the Medical Field Units. The objective was to extend its activities to all rural areas of the country, and to widen its scope to include as many endemic diseases as possible.[1] For its entire period of operation, the MFU became known among rural communities as "Campaign." As already noted, the MFUs were also responsible for epidemic disease control. Additional tasks of the Units were to conduct a general survey in the field of endemic disease, and to treat in the field all diseases for which satisfactory remedies were available in such circumstances. The broad scope given the MFU required the recruitment and deployment of several categories of staff in the field.

[1] B.B. Waddy. 'Organisation and Work of the Gold Coast Medical Field Units'. Report on Ordinary Meeting of the Royal Society of Tropical Medicine and Hygiene held at Manson House, 26, Portland Place, London, on Thursday, 17th May, 1956.

3.2 Categories of Staff Working with Medical Field Units

In order to be able to operate efficiently, the MFU employed categories of staff with varied expertise. There were four categories of staff: Senior Staff, Junior Staff, Clerical Staff, and daily-paid non-technical staff.

3.2.1 Senior Staff

The Medical Field Units were organised into arbitrary territorial regions. Each region at least required a staff member of the Senior category. The chart below provides details of the categories of Senior Staff who were employed by the MFU.

From the figure below (Fig. 3.1.) it is evident that the Medical Officers and the Field Superintendents formed the bulk of the Senior Staff category. The rationale for this was a gradual shift in the policy of the colonial bureaucracy involving health and health practice in the Gold Coast Colony. The shift was part of the general concern expressed in London about issues of health in the colonies. For example in a famous dispatch of May 1898, Joseph Chamberlain enunciated the principle of common responsibility, equally incumbent upon all colonial administrations and shared by the Imperial Government, for the reduction of the mortality of Europeans and Africans in the tropical Colonies and Dependencies, and to that end undertook the provision of a specially trained personnel for medical services overseas.[2] This policy contributed to the provision, at that time, of an adequate number of medical officers and field superintendents. The presence of other equally important groups such as reclamation officers, entomologists, and regional field supervisors, was due to the fact that tropical medicine and the outbreak of epidemics demanded a far wider field, both for research, practice, prevention, and treatment. Figure 3.1 provides details regarding the categories of Senior Staff that were engaged in the MFU. They include: BI-Biologist, DO- Development Officer, ET-Entomologist, FS-Field Superintendent, LS-Laboratory Superintendent, MO-Medical

[2] The Colonial Medical Service. *The British Medical Journal*, Vol. 2, No. 3678 (Jul. 4, 1931), pp. 11e–17e.

Officers, MSS-Medical Store Superintendent, RFS-Regional Field Supervisors, RO-Reclamation Officer, SE-Special Entomologist, SEO-Senior Executive Officer, and TCO-Tsetse Control Officer.

It is important to highlight a few things in the chart regarding the recruitment of a high number of Field Superintendents and Medical Officers. Both the Field Superintendent and the Medical Officer played complementary roles in the Medical Field Units. The Medical Officers were directly responsible for the treatment. The Field Superintendents exercised oversight responsibilities over resource allocation—human, financial, materials, and supervision among others. The recruitment of biologists and entomologists into the MFU was to ensure that vector-borne diseases were well identified, and that it developed the necessary tools for prevention, control, and treatment. The development officers usually connected and coordinated the activities of the various stakeholders such as the technicians, medical officers, and the community. Their role was key in ensuring the smooth operations of the MFU in any given community.

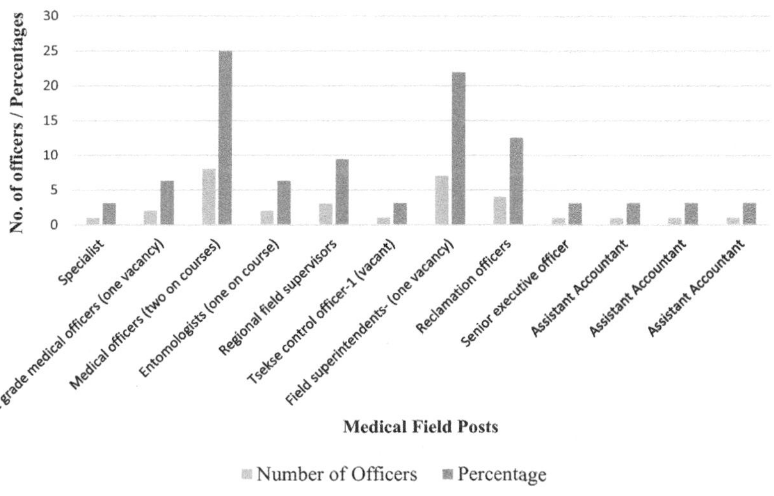

Fig. 3.1 MFU: Senior staff (1960/61)

3.2.2 *Junior Staff*

Just as occurred among the Senior Staff, the Junior Staff also had different categories of staff as represented in Fig. 3.2 below. The divisions include: FAG I-Field Assistant Grade I, FAG II-Field Assistant Grade II, FTE-Field Technician Established, FT U-Field Technician Unestablished, RU-Recorders Unestablished, and TCS-Tsetse Control.

The Junior Staff category as represented in Fig. 3.2 was considered critical to the operation of the Medical Field Units. Junior Staff comprised Field Assistant Grade I, Field Assistant Grade II, Field Technician Established, Field Technician Unestablished, Recorders Unestablished, Tsetse Control Staff, and Trainees.

Unlike the Senior Staff who were mostly expatriates, the Junior Staff were mostly from the indigenous population of the Gold Coast. They had the responsibility of carrying out administrative and clinical tasks during field visits. Without them the work of the Medical Officers and Field Superintendents, in spite of their specialisation, could not function very well in practice. The Junior Staff had the duty of facilitating a wide range

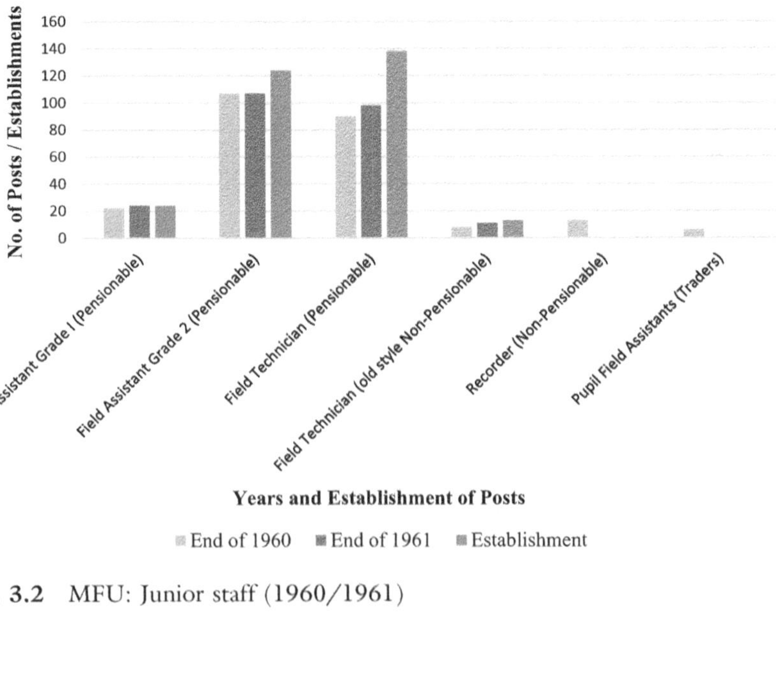

Fig. 3.2 MFU: Junior staff (1960/1961)

of standardised tasks to enable Senior Staff to perform more complex tasks. Within the Junior Staff there existed a binary in terms of qualified versus unqualified, or professionally qualified versus the support workforce. Field Assistants were classified under the qualified category, and so were the established field technicians and recorders. Technicians are persons who have the scientific knowledge and necessary competencies in some recognised branch of science to support the work of professional scientists or engineers (Anold, 1965). In the chart below, the category "unestablished" technicians, represented as "U," were usually in training, and yet to qualify as Technicians. Essentially the categorisation of established and unestablished reveals the nature of the skill mix in the Junior Staff category, which created some boundaries between the staff and the types and levels of work that was performed in the field. From the table it was obvious that there was a higher recruitment of Field Assistants FAG II-Field Assistant Grade II and FTE-Field Technician Established, between 1960 and 1961.

The general understanding is that the increase in "Established Technicians" was due to several factors, including a substantial pool of ex-servicemen who were willing to take up an appointment with the health sector at the time, and the general expansion of the civil and health sector at that time, which fell in line with Nkrumah's vision of modernising and developing the health sector. For purposes of comparison, by 1953 approximately ninety percent of all hospitals were in the south, and the population of beds per person was 478:1 in the south, but 35,000:1 in the north (Anyinam, 1989). The field units were considered an important extension and addition to the health infrastructure in the north, even though their focus was on epidemiology.

3.2.3 Clerical Staff

The employment of clerks represented in Fig. 3.3 (consisting of CA-Clerical Assistants, CO-Clerical Officer, EO-Executive Officers, SG-Stenographer, TY-Typist) became necessary when the administration of the Medical Field Units decided to have an entirely new section for typing and storing data, separate from doctors and technicians whose duty it was to identify and treat diseases. The clerical unit became more important when Kintampo was formally made the administrative capital of all the Medical Field Units. Kintampo is located in the middle of Ghana. Due to its unique location, logistics could easily be deployed from there.

Such activities required mostly administrative and clerical personnel who dealt with most urgent administrative and logistical matters (Addae, 1997, p. 114). Even though they were all classified as clerical staff, their duties varied. For example, the clerical assistant was responsible for filing reports, and providing and ensuring the smooth flow of communication, such as the despatch and receiving of letters and telegraphic messages. Clerical assistants are a step below the clerical officer, who work directly with the medical and technical staff. The executive officers were responsible for the planning, direction, and coordination of the daily operations of the Medical Field Units. The typists in the Medical Field Units were responsible for typing out documents and letters. In some cases, where there were no clerical assistants, the typists also performed other duties such as filing, printing, and copying documents, along with answering the phones. In the 1960s, the five regional centres and about thirteen permanent bases all had stores, which meant a greater dependence on the clerical staff.

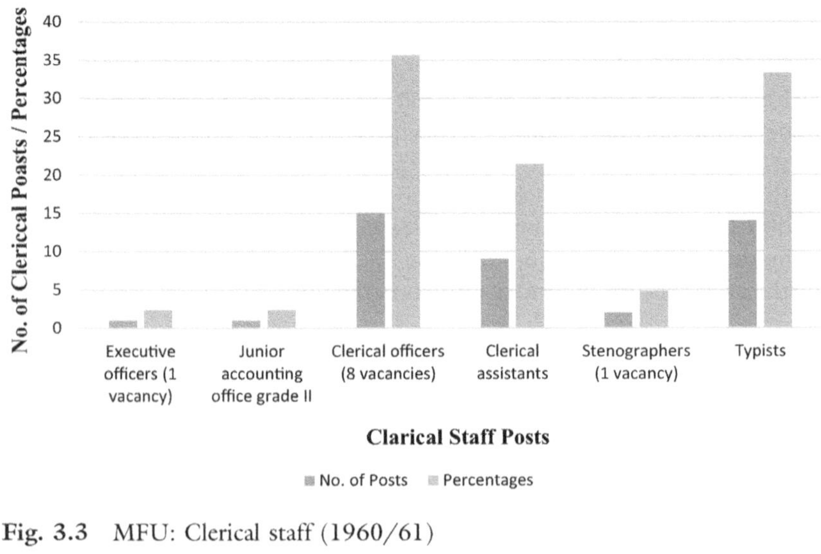

Fig. 3.3 MFU: Clerical staff (1960/61)

3.2.4 Non-technical Staff

The fulcrum on which the wheel of Medical Field Unit rotated was those below the Junior Staff, sometimes with little or no Western education. As noted in Fig. 3.4 below, they consist of the following: DR-Drivers, HE-Headmen, PL&C,M,W-Permanent Laborers & Carriers, Messengers, Watchman, and TR-Tradesmen.

It is important to single out for discussion the issue of carriers and drivers in the transport section of the MFU, as well as labourers, since they compose quite a big category in the chart above. As already noted, the activities of the MFU required constant movement of personnel and goods. Three modes of transport were utilised in that regard: head portage carriers, cycle-based transport—bicycles and motor bikes—and other motor vehicles. Regarding head-load porters, or carriers, three types were distinguishable within the period under review. There were those who carried loads, staff, and their dependents.

Awedoba, a professor of medical anthropology at the University of Ghana, recalls his experience as follows:

> I was born in the 1950s and I still have very good memories about the activities of the Medical Field Unit. My father was an ex-service man and

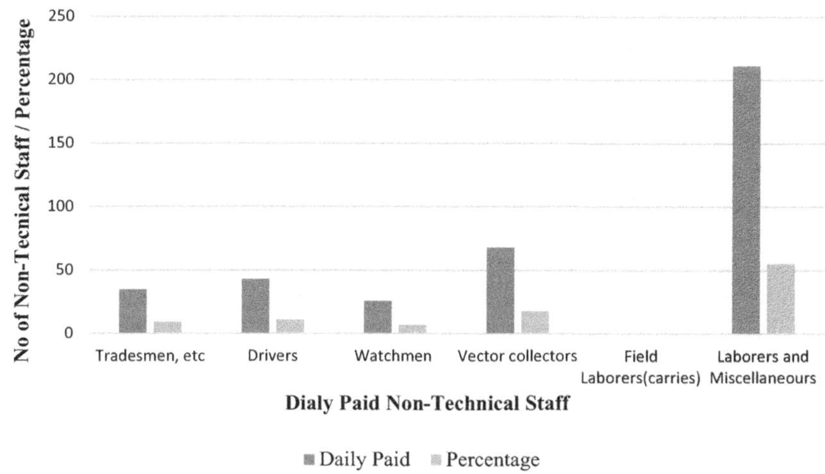

Fig. 3.4 MFU: Daily-paid non-technical staff (1960/61)

> he was recruited to work with the Unit after his disbandment from the military. I remember being carried on the shoulders by a carrier and the rest carried my father's medical equipment and other logistics. The head porters were very important.[3]

The porters described above had a kind of permanent attachment to the MFU and their staff. Others were freelance carriers. The freelance carriers were usually seasonal labour migrants who from time to time moved to the southern part of Ghana in order to work and to earn money. Since some of them went by foot they were easily identified, and were offered carriage jobs, to carry medical supplies, equipment, or personnel. It is important to indicate that the utilisation of carriers, some of whom may have been from the very area where epidemics may have broken out, was a useful adaptation to the unequal geographical knowledge of the medical team in the area of operation. Since beyond carriage, carriers also served as guides to the medical team, they played an important role in facilitating access to basic but important logistics such as accommodation and food.

In order to ensure that there was efficiency, the position of headman was created in the non-technical staff category. The Headman or Headmen were called the *harrman* (corrupted from headman) by the non-technical staff. The *harrman* would have been employed earlier and have a sound working knowledge of the Medical Field Units, particularly of the movement of staff and logistics. It was the *harrman's* duty to mobilise the workers under him to execute any kind of assignment that was given by those in the technical category.

Apart from portage, other forms of transport were also utilised in the field by the Medical Field Units. They made use of bicycles, motorcycles, and other vehicles. As of 1958 the Medical Field Units had 12 Range Rovers, three five-ton trucks, six three-ton trucks, 11 one-and-a-half-ton trucks, and five crew cars. In total the Medical Field Units had 37 of its own vehicles. The United Nations International Children's Fund also supplied 12 Range Rovers and one two-ton truck. In total the MFU had 50 vehicles in 1958.[4] It is important to point out that not all the vehicles were in very good condition, and therefore not on the road. That

[3] Interview with Professor Albert Awedoba at the Institute of African Studies on 29th November, 2022.

[4] Ghana Medical Field Units Annual Report 1958.

might explain the number of drivers at less than fifty in the bar chart above (Fig. 3.4). Field staff were also given pedal cycles and Teagle Jet motorcycles. Later, due to their inefficiency, the Teagle Jet motorcycles were replaced with NSU motorcycles. Among all the modes of transport used by the Medical Field Units, it was the bicycles that lasted the longest. Porters easily deserted. Vehicles were rendered useless in areas where there were no roads, and the unmotorable nature of the roads in the rural areas also drove the maintenance cost of motor vehicles higher. Bicycles had several advantages. The flat nature of the environment where the field units operated made their use easy. Also, the fact that bicycles had a less complex operational and mechanical system as compared to cars and motorcycles, as well as a lower maintenance cost, and the availability of several bicycle fitters in the field of operation of Medical Field Units, all ensured a longer life span of bicycles in the field.

Labourers and messengers were usually in charge of the maintenance of the premises of the field units. Some labourers were also responsible for clearing vegetation around rivers, streams, and swamps. Their role was critical as they provided a safety belt around water systems which served as breeding grounds for tsetse flies, which were important vectors in the transmission of sleeping sickness to human beings. Writing about fly eradication and epidemics in the Gold Coast, Jeff D. Grischow (2006, p. 382) notes:

> A major trypanosomiasis pandemic hit the Gold Coast and the colonial administration invited Morris back to the colony. He returned in 1937, keen to revive his anti-tsetse work. By this time, Morris's method of choice was a variation on the bush-clearing model called 'discriminative' or 'selective' clearing, which targeted specific plant associations along river banks in core trypanosomiasis areas. This approach reflected the belief that tsetse flies retreated to restricted habitats along river banks during the dry season. Clearing those habitats would eradicate the flies and eliminate the disease.

In essence, all the categories of MFU staff mentioned above including Senior Staff, Junior Staff, Clerical Staff, and non-technical staff played a critical role in the management and functioning of the Medical Field Units. As Waddy (1956, p. 316) noted:

> Doctors being so scarce, the lay auxiliaries play a most important part in the work. They are graded as follows. Ranking as senior civil servants are Regional Field Supervisors and Field Superintendents, the former being

> sometimes Europeans with wide field experience; most in both ranks are Africans who have, essentially, advanced through the ranks of Medical Field Units and have shown outstanding ability in all aspects of the work. Ranking as junior permanent civil servants are Field Assistants in two grades. The daily-paid rank and file are Technicians. Those of under three years' service rank as pupil Field Assistants. At the end of their training, if successful, they become Field Assistants; if of lower ability they become Technicians. This ranking is an adaptation of the original Trypanosomiasis Campaign system, under which many of the Technicians were illiterate...to describe the part played by these men it is easiest to begin at the front line of field medicine, the work of a present day survey team.

The quote above emphasises coordination as an important element in handling epidemics and diseases.

3.2.5 Some General Comments on the Operations of MFU

The main duty of the MFU was to control epidemics and immediately respond to outbreaks. Their field of operation included diseases such as smallpox, sleeping sickness, and Cerebrospinal meningitis (CSM), among others. But it was sleeping sickness, CSM, and yaws that the Units gave considerable attention. The addition of the latter was because of the combined efforts of the World Health Organization and the United Nations Children's Fund, which assisted the campaign against yaws as part of a single plan of operation for northern Ghana and Volta Togoland.

As a rule, Medical Officers appointed from Britain to the Gold Coast, including those assigned to work with the MFU, were required upon their appointment to undergo a three months course of instruction at the London or Liverpool School of Tropical Medicine, and to obtain a certificate of proficiency before taking up their appointment. But the basic training given to trainees in the MFU was always in the field. The trainee received experience in different aspects of the work of a field team, such as census taking, microscopy, vaccination, and selection, that is naked-eye diagnosis of various infections such as yaws, and injection techniques, among others. After a sufficient period, formal tests are carried out and he or she is qualified as competent to perform some or all of the different duties as a team member in the MFU.[5]

[5] Ghana Medical Field Units Annual Report 1958.

The core operation areas of the Medical Field Units were in the northern parts of Ghana but there were other satellite operational areas that were established in other parts of Ghana. In all the Units had about five key headquarters in Ghana. In North East, the headquarters was in Gambaga. In Northwest, the Headquarters was in Wa. In Ashanti, the headquarters was in Kintampo. In the Transvolta Togoland, the Headquarters was in Ho, and in the Eastern Region the Headquarters was in Koforidua. In addition to the five headquarters in the regions mentioned above, there were additional thirteen Treatment Centres that were established in 1961. Two specialist Units were also set up. The first was called the Simulium Control Unit, and the second was the Tsetse Control Unit.

It was from the operational capitals or "regional capitals" of Gambaga, Wa, Kintampo, Koforidua, and Ho that the staff branched out to areas far beyond such as Tamale, Yendi, Kpandai, Lawra, Kumasi, Accra, and several rural areas, to handle epidemics and other diseases. The officer in charge of a region had at his disposal, for routine field survey, normally two groups each consisting of two (though sometimes only one) survey teams, and treatment teams. Surveying was an important aspect of the work of the MFU, as the chart in Fig. 3.5 shows. Indeed, much of the work of MFU depended on this kind of precise generation of data on diseases and people. This point was stressed further in the report of the Medical Field Units in 1958. The report indicates:

> Although the greatest field efforts in 1958 have been against yaws, sleeping sickness and cerebrospinal meningitis, an important work of the MFU continuous to be the collection of data regarding endemic diseases by the use of survey teams. This information requires to be assessed and a statistical branch in Headquarters is essential; only slowly can this be built up.[6]

Surveys are important because geographically precise identification and targeting of populations at risk of vaccine-preventable diseases constitute a potentially useful evidence base to evaluate the performance of vaccination strategies. These estimates are also valuable for identifying missed communities, hence enabling targeted interventions and better resource allocation (Utazi et al., 2023).

[6] Ghana Field Unit Annual Report 1958.

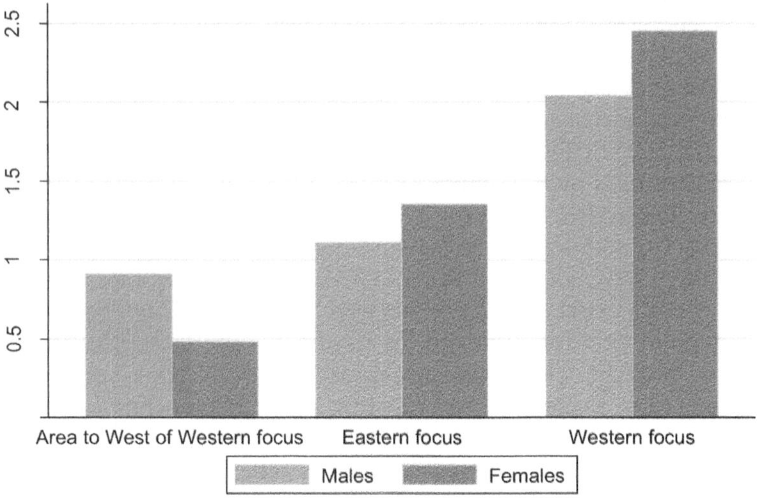

Fig. 3.5 Incidence of sleeping sickness in males and females

This is even more important in the activities of MFU as treatment teams in addition to the survey teams must work hand in hand. The allocation of treatment teams depended on the local endemic levels of diseases requiring intravenous therapy. They consisted of only two men and probably a carrier or two, and could be formed as the need arose; occasionally a survey team would be temporarily broken up into treatment teams to finish off the work in an area after completing its survey. Usually a treatment team deals with only one disease at a time. Its weekly round might include three or four villages several miles apart.

As indicated, the initial conceptualisation of the Medical Field Units was for them to operate in the northern part of the country where there were endemic problems of sleeping sickness. The concentration in these areas was due to the fact that although sleeping sickness dates from the nineteenth century in the Gold Coast, colonial officials expressed little concern until reports of sleeping sickness escalated in the mid-1920s from the Lawra (Western Focus) and Mamprusi districts of the Northern Territories (Grischow, 2006, p. 384).

Reported incidences in Mamprusi became high as compared to other areas because the headquarters of MFU was stationed in Gambaga, the capital of the Mamprusi area.[7] Furthermore Mamprusi was among the first places where the disease was discovered. Even though the population of those surveyed in western and eastern parts of the north was lower as compared to Mamprusi, there were more epidemic cases recorded by the MFU in the western part of the north, as evidenced in the bar chart in Fig. 3.5. The reason is that the Sisili river was one of the major rivers of north-western Ghana, along with the Black Volta and Kulpawn rivers that housed a lot of tsetse flies, and they were all located in the northwest. In Fig. 3.5, surveys by the MFU also revealed that the same area had a high incidence of male-to-female infections, with female infections being higher in both the east and the west. The high rate of infections among women is reflective of the occupations in the area, with women having the extra burden of fetching water and firewood in addition to farming. These activities usually exposed them more than males, as the farm and riverine areas experienced a heavy infestation of tsetse flies. The figures of the west of Western Focus fall in the areas of Nandom and Hamile; these are areas that have fewer water systems and are a bit dry, thereby reducing the incidence of tsetse infestation.

In essence, the Medical Field Units were established to handle diseases. The Units were very successful in plotting certain endemic diseases during field surveys, as the example of sleeping sickness shows in the charts provided above. Staff of the MFU also provided treatment to communities affected by diseases. The Medical Field Units became one of the most efficient instruments of medical services in combating some of the endemic diseases in Ghana. The eradication of yaws; the control of trypanosomiasis; their participation in smallpox vaccination and leprosy finding; their role in medication and early case findings and treatment of CSM; and their epidemiological surveys of several other endemic diseases, made the MFU a unique medical entity (Addae, 1997). The immense role played by the Medical Field Units in rural health cannot be overstated especially when health centres were mostly situated in the southern coastal regions, with three hospitals located in the colonial capital of Accra. However, their success also came with some problems. The next section of this chapter discusses the problems that arose in the operations of the MFU in Ghana.

[7] In terms of operations of MFU Gambaga not Nalerigu was considered the capital. For several years during the colonial period Gambaga had served as the capital for the Northern Territory.

3.3 Problems

The MFU had a shortage of medical staff, which was evident in their operations. For the whole Unit there were ten doctors in 1961, of whom four were Ghanaian and six were European. Out of the ten, two had gone abroad to undertake further studies as of 1961. Due to insufficient staff, it was the policy of the Units to accept the responsibility of dropping whatever they were doing to take control of any major epidemic outside of their area of operations. The fact that routine vaccinations were also added to their duties meant that the staff were at all times thinly distributed and overburdened. A comment on the staffing situation in the 1950s is worth repeating here:

> But in MFU for several years now trainees have constituted an extremely large and important element more than thirty percent of the staff to carry out technical work... the staffing situation in the Simulium Control Unit, MFU stores and other special branches illustrate the difficulty. Some of the older and trained persons in MFU, junior technical grade are not available for posting.[8]

Sometimes staff resorted to ad hoc mass vaccination campaign when there were outbreaks. Furthermore, in order to lessen the pressure, staff of the MFU at times had to recruit local temporary staff on the spot, and provide some training for them, to be able to elicit clinical information related to specific diseases. Such a plan often leads to misdiagnosis. In order to save time and energy involved in visiting villages, staff often visited markets and carried out surveys and examinations of persons in the market. Such a medical methodology had the defect of cutting out a crucial segment of the population since there was the likelihood of only healthy people visiting the markets, while the sick may likely stay home.[9]

The second problem associated with the MFU was infrastructure and logistics. As already indicated, data generation was very key to the functioning of the MFU. In order to generate data, surveys would have to be conducted. Incidentally, at the time of their operations, there were few motorable roads. Most of the areas were inaccessible due to rivers,

[8] Ghana Medical Field Units Annual Report 1958.

[9] B.B. Waddy. 'Organisation and Work of the Gold Coast Medical Field Units'. Report on Ordinary Meeting of the Royal Society of Tropical Medicine and Hygiene held at Manson House, 26, Portland Place, London, on Thursday, 17th May, 1956.

streams, and tree cover. Such difficulties led to the coinage of the terminology "overseas settlements" –referring to the inaccessible areas at the time of operation of the MFU. In addition, there were few vehicles at the disposal of the staff. Most of them had to either walk or ride bicycles. Such modes of transport proved to be useful but at the same time tiresome. The additional problem had to do with the transmission of data to the headquarters in Kintampo, following Kintampo's designation as administrative capital. As a result of distance, up-to-date data could not be provided, as sometimes surveys conducted the previous month only arrived in Kintampo the next month due to the slow pace of mail delivery. This often compelled Medical Officers to leave their area of operation and carry the data collected to Kintampo. Such actions revealed the importance of data production, which was possibly as important as the treatment of people.

In most rural areas the MFU staff had no bungalows to stay in. In most cases it was the chief of the village who had to make arrangements in his compound or appeal to other members of the community to provide accommodation to staff who came to perform official duties. In some of the well-established towns, staff usually rented accommodation from house owners. In order to begin work, sometimes school buildings were taken over or huts were constructed using guinea corn or sorghum stock. Such huts served as places for the dispensation of medication as well as "admission rooms." The infrastructural difficulties often led to some resignations by the staff of MFU. An informant points out that since the possibility of resignation was very high, usually ex-servicemen were preferred during recruitment of field technicians, since they mostly went beyond the call for duty to stay at post no matter the circumstances.

Mile-long clearance of bushes, shrubs, and trees around villages, along the roads, and on water systems was an essential component of the activities of the MFU, especially during severe outbreaks. The fact that there were several rivers and streams in their area of operation meant that the cost of clearance went very high. For example, it was reported that in 1958 about one hundred and twenty seven pounds was spent per mile.[10] As a result, in some cases the targeted clearing quotas were not met.

The overconcentration of activities in the northern part of the country meant that other more severely affected areas in the south only received

[10] Ghana Medical Field Units Annual Report 1958.

ad hoc attention. For example, on the blind side of the MFU, epidemic situations had picked up in Ashanti in the 1950s, a situation which might have been avoided had the activities of MFU been evenly distributed around the country. Polyvalent Surveys for sleeping sickness in communities in Ashanti had shown the highest rates of infections along the roads. This should have been expected considering that Ashanti relied heavily on migrant labour from the north who mostly worked on cocoa farms and in the mines, and most of whom came by foot. Also, the cattle trade between the north and Ashanti was very vibrant, and most of the cattle were driven down south through Yeji to Ashanti, thus accounting for the transmission of such endemic situations into Ashanti. Finally, because of concentration in the north, the MFU was not operational in the Western and Central Regions of Ghana even though an office, a treatment centre, and other buildings of the Unit's headquarters at Tarkwa were completed, and work on a doctors' house had begun in 1961.

3.4 Conclusion

The original Trypanosomiases Campaign had been formed in Gambaga in 1937. It comprised about thirty staff who were for the most part locally recruited in Mamprusi. They were trained in elementary microscopy, and in the simple record-keeping and census-taking that mass control of sleeping sickness demands. In the 1940s following the reduction of epidemic cases, governments sought to convert their monovalent sleeping sickness organisations into polyvalent services which would extend their work to the control of other diseases. The principles required to control diseases occasioned the employment of several categories of staff, as indicated in the charts above, to be able to ascertain cases of infection through large-scale examination of entire populations within affected areas, and to eradicate or control through the mass treatment of cases.

Essentially, from the 1940s to the 1960s the activities of the MFU centred on critical areas that required the control of particular communicable diseases using specific rather than general measures for the attack of such diseases. The control mechanisms deployed included the destruction of reservoirs of infection of diseases, or immediate eradication of the intermediate host and provision of specific protection through vaccination or chemoprophylaxis for each member of the community exposed to the disease. The MFU was also to assess the vast amount of information on disease behaviour collected by the survey teams in the field and to analyse the results of the various disease control measures. Detailed records were made on infections such as yaws and sleeping sickness, as well as on treated cases and the control mechanisms used to combat endemic conditions.[11] The data was collected in such a way that it could best be used to help define the geographical and demographical patterns of the separate diseases, and to indicate the trends in their prevalence. Such information assisted in planning future control programmes for endemic and epidemic diseases. Finally, the MFU became that body that was constantly in readiness to respond to emergency epidemic conditions, as they were a highly mobile unit. Ultimately, following the overhauls of the medical system in Ghana at the beginning of the 1970s, activities of the MFU came to an end. The Unit was transformed into the Rural Health Services, and now it counts as the Epidemiology Unit of the Ghana health service.

Conflict of Interest No conflict of interest is declared.

References

Addae, S. (1997). *History of western medicine in Ghana 1880–1960*. Durham Academic Press.

Anold, W. M. (1965). The federal government's role in the training of technicians. *Research Management, 8*(6), 369–381.

Anyinam, C. A. (1989). The social costs of the International Monetary Fund's Adjustment Programs for poverty: The case of Health Care Development in Ghana. *International Journal of Health Services, 19*(3), 531–547.

Bodenheimer, T. S. (1969). Mobile units: A solution to the rural health problem? *Medical Care, 7*(2), 144–154.

Grischow, J. D. (2006). K. R. S. Morris and Tsetse Eradication in the Gold Coast, 1928-51. *Africa, 76*(3), 381–401.

Mengistu, D., & Misganaw, E. (2006). *Community Health Nursing: Ethiopia Public Health Training Initiative*. University of Gondar.

Ntewusu, S. A. (2014). Serendipity: Conducting research on social history in Ghana's archives. *History in Africa, 41*, 417–423.

Scott, D. (1962, September). The history and work of the medical field units in Ghana. *Ghana Medical Journal*, 19–21.

Utazi, C. E., Aheto, J., Wigley, A., Tejedor-Garavito, N., Bonnie, A., Nnanatu, C., Wagai, J., Williams, C., Setayesh, H., Tatem, A., & Cutts, F. (2023).

[11] Medical Field Units Annual Report, 1961.

Mapping the distribution of zero-dose children to assess the performance of vaccine delivery strategies and their relationships with measles incidence in Nigeria. *Vaccine, 41*(1), 170–181.
Waddy, B. B. (1956). The organisation and work of the Gold Coast Medical Field Units. *Transactions of the Royal Society of Tropical Medicine and Hygiene, 50*(4), 313–343.

PART II

Ethnographies of the Health Register

CHAPTER 4

Mental Health in Ghana: Standardisation, Advocacy and Changing Perceptions of Care and Disease

Humphrey Asamoah Agyekum

4.1 Introduction: The Ghanaian Relationship to Mental Health

Ghanaians have a complex relationship with mental health and those suffering from mental disorders. Officially, mental health in Ghana is defined as "a condition of the mind in which there is a clinically significant disturbance of mental or behavioural functioning associated with distress, or interference of daily life and manifesting as disturbance of speech, perception, mood, thought, volition, orientation, or other cognitive functions to such a degree as to be considered pathological but excludes social

No conflict of interest is declared.

H. A. Agyekum (✉)
University of Copenhagen, Copenhagen, Denmark
e-mail: haa@anthro.ku.dk

A. Thiel and S. A. Ntewusu (eds.), *The Social Life of Health Data*,
https://doi.org/10.1007/978-981-97-3500-6_4

deviance without personal dysfunction" (cf. Badu et al., 2018; Government of Ghana, 2012; Walker & Osei, 2017). In other words, at the governmental level, mental health is considered a medical condition based on internationally recognised standardised mental health symptoms (see this chapter's discussion of DSM-5 below). Standardisation of protocols (Lampland & Star, 2009) is aligned with a logic of testing and evidence in medical decision-making. Beisel et al. (2018) have described this standardisation as a stock of knowledge that seeks to validate what is already known or suspected, but which does not lend itself to engaging with other forms of knowing. Yet, for ordinary Ghanaians, mental health is a sensitive issue associated with the supranatural realm (Lauterbach, 2010; Meyer, 2012), rather than with standard medical classifications.

A core assumption in Ghana's mental health system is that limited knowledge about mental health diagnoses—but also about specific treatment approaches[1]—does not allow people suffering from mental illness to seek a systematic evaluation of the efficacy of clinical treatment (Arias et al., 2016), leading sufferers to consult traditional and faith-based healing systems and pathways instead (Nortje et al., 2016; Rathod et al., 2017). Patients meanwhile associate clinical institutions with the danger of infection, rather than seeing them as facilities of care. This chapter details the work of Ghanaian mental health providers who seek to transform societal perspectives on mental health and care in Ghana through implementation, use, and dissemination of international standard protocols such as the DSM-5. The chapter positions itself in medical anthropology, and analyses mental health care in Ghana through the lens of socio-cultural conditions and the human dimensions of health (Mhlanga, 2023). Medical anthropology is not only interested in investigating experiences of human health and healthcare systems, but also treatments of illness (Mhlanga, 2023). Taking the specific perspective of mental health professionals and their engagement in advocacy, the chapter discusses how standardisation intersects with changing perceptions of mental health and care in Ghana.

Many studies to date have examined the state of mental health care in Ghana in its various facets. Generally, research initially focused on clinical

[1] Ghanaians' limited appreciation of mental health as a clinical condition has various reasons, ranging from colonial authorities' preference for a biomedical approach to mental disorders to cultural beliefs, as will be discussed throughout this chapter (Kpobi et al., 2023).

case reports and psychiatric epidemiological studies (Adomakoh, 1972a, 1972b, Foster & Ingram, 1962, Turkson & Dua, 1996, Asare, 2001). The studies in this period focused on the biomedical aspects of mental health, but also on the prevalence of psychiatric conditions, and the manifestation thereof in hospitals and communities. Over the last two decades, mental health research in Ghana has explored the state of mental health provisions and services (Kpobi et al., 2023, Read & Doku, 2012), but also more specific aspects of resource utilisation (Adika et al., 2017; Awenva et al., 2010), the cultural appropriateness of measures, or stigma, and lay beliefs about conditions such as depression (cf. for instance Anum et al., 2020; Eshun et al., 1998; Walters et al., 1999), substance abuse (Affinnih, 2005), suicidal behaviour (cf. Eshun, 2000; Hjelmeland et al., 2008), and schizophrenia (Field, 1958, 1960; Turkson, 2000).

This chapter contributes to this body of research through the medical anthropological examination of socio-cultural constructions and perceptions of mental health in Ghana, and specifically the role of standards in the effort to change harmful perceptions of mental health. It will be argued here that there is a concerted effort driven by both local and foreign-trained mental health professionals to alter perceptions of the phenomenon. Mental health professionals do so through the mobilisation of standardised protocols in the mental health sector, such as the Diagnostic and Statistical Manual of Mental Disorders, Fifth Edition, Text Revision (DSM-5-TR), in clinical practices, advocacy, and education initiatives in Ghanaian mass media outlets. However, social dynamics of illness and care intersect with standardising forces in complex ways. The chapter proceeds by detailing the challenges of mental health care in Ghana, before focusing on the work of standardisation in the contexts of advocacy and education.

Fieldwork for this study was undertaken between June and December 2017 in Accra, Ghana. During the fieldwork, interviews were conducted with twelve psychologists. The interactions took the form of informal conversations and semi-structured interviews, lasting between thirty minutes and an hour and a half. Of the twelve psychologists interviewed for the present study, ten were trained at American, Canadian, and British universities, while two were trained in Ghana for their graduate, doctorate, or post-doctorate education. The clinicians interviewed varied in age from thirty to fifty-five years, and had begun their careers in the 1990s up to the present.

4.2 Challenges of Mental Health Care

Mental health care in Ghana is fraught with multiple societal, political, and infrastructural challenges. This section details the multiple factors contributing to the negative perceptions of mental health in Ghana, and the associated challenges for mental health advocacy.

4.2.1 Low Policy Priority and Underinvestment

Mental health in Ghana is constrained by its low political priority. The issue's absence from the public agenda contributes to it being poorly understood as a medical phenomenon in Ghanaian society (Omar et al., 2010). Up to 2012, Ghanaian policymakers were not overly concerned with mental health care, resulting in a lack of up-to-date mental health legislation. In the words of a psychologist, this can be attributed to historical antecedents: "Mental health in Ghana is the backbencher of health care. In its formative years, there was no policy concerning mental health issues."[2] Notably, the enactment of the Asylum Ordinance in 1888 by the then Governor of the Gold Coast, Sir Griffith Edwards, criminalised insanity, to the effect that mentally ill people were imprisoned rather than cared for (cf. Adu-Gyamfi, 2017; Fournier, 2012). Those suffering from mental illness were considered dangerous deviants who would be jailed, or physically restrained due to the then-prevalent fear of them becoming a societal risk. This laid the groundwork for how mental health would be treated and assessed for generations to come; the colonial approach of confining patients persists to the present in psychiatric hospitals, prayer camps, or in patients' homes (cf. Adu-Gyamfi, 2017; Fournier, 2012).

Continuous lack of policy priority has resulted in structural difficulties in mental health service provision.[3] The World Health Organization (WHO) estimates that 25% of the world's population will suffer from mental, behavioural, or neurological disorders, such as schizophrenia, mental retardation, and stress-related disorders, during their lifetime (Fournier, 2012). The Ghana Health Service, the body responsible for

[2] Interview with Dr. W., 37 Military Hospital, Accra, Ghana (November 2017).

[3] However, Ghana has announced that from 2024 mental health will be included in the benefit package of the National Health Insurance Scheme.

implementing the country's healthcare policies and enforcing clinical standards, estimated that around 21% of adult Ghanaians experience moderate or severe psychological distress at any time (Canavan et al., 2016).

Yet, the vast majority of the Ghanaian population has little or no access to mental health services. Ghana has three main mental health public hospitals: Accra Psychiatric Hospital, Pantang Hospital, and Ankaful Psychiatric Hospital; all located in the south of the country (Fournier, 2012). In addition, facilities are challenged by the absence or irregular supply of essential medications, such as antipsychotics, anxiolytics, antidepressants, and mood stabilisers (Adu-Gyamfi, 2017, Badu et al., 2018, see also Ofori-Atta et al., 2010). As a result, those suffering from mental disorders cannot be treated adequately, which results in patients behaving absent-mindedly, violently, or erratically, which likely perpetuates harmful societal perceptions of patients and mental illness in general.[4]

For these reasons, when Ghana passed the Mental Health Act in 2012, it was hoped that it would create a new mental health system with improved access and new attention to the rights[5] of patients (Walker & Osei, 2017). The 2012 law included provisions for the creation of a modern, community-based mental health system (Walker & Osei, 2017), a novelty in Ghana's mental health care system. Small psychiatric units were set up at regional, district, and community hospitals and clinics in previously underserved regions of the country, including in the rural central and northern belt (Kpobi et al., 2023). Yet, although there were "more units springing up all over the country,"[6] and the expansion resulted in a growth in community mental health, with the deployment of hundreds of community mental health workers to health facilities across Ghana (Kpobi et al., 2023), problems of underinvestment in infrastructure and personnel still plague the mental health sector.

Like many low-income post-colonial countries in Africa, Ghana's population since independence in 1957 has expanded more than fivefold, which also means growth in the numbers of people suffering from mental

[4] The 1972 Mental Health Decree (NRCD 30) which sought to replace these laws was never implemented (Doku et al, 2012; Osei et al., 2011), and hence did little to change the existing negative perceptions surrounding mental health in Ghana.

[5] As a result of the history of harmful mental health legislation in the West African country and colonial era laws, the rights of patients could in the past be abused without repercussions for the abuser, as there were no legal protections for patients.

[6] Interview with Dr. B-O., Accra, Ghana (July 2017).

disorders. Meanwhile, Ghana has not developed the infrastructure and public services, including mental health care, to keep pace with population growth (Ofori-Atta et al., 2010). As a result, there is not only a persistent lack of investment in the mental health infrastructure, but also in personnel. Ghanaian mental health professionals have unattractive working conditions. Many express job dissatisfaction and a desire to seek better job opportunities either abroad or outside the mental health sector (Badu et al., 2018). Ghana, like many countries on the continent, has fewer than one psychiatrist per 100,000 people, while seventy percent of African countries allocate the mental health sector less than 1% of the total health budget (Fournier, 2012). Consequently the doctor-patient ratio is one psychiatrist per 1.5 million people (Fournier, 2012). The dire lack of mental health professionals in Ghana also stems from the breakdown of those who graduated from health training institutions: in 2005, approximately 190 medical doctors graduated, but none was specialised in psychology or psychiatry (Ofori-Atta et al., 2010).

In other words, since the colonial period, there has been a consistent lack of investment in mental health infrastructure and personnel. The lack of investment in infrastructure and personnel means that those suffering from mental illness do not receive the necessary care, even if professionals want to offer them care based on the standardised protocols, such as the DSM-5. The lack of legislation for the mental health sector has also for many decades shaped not only how the system is financed and structured, but also how the sector is experienced and viewed by the Ghanaian public. The low morale of mental health professionals, and the low quality of service provision, all play into the already negative societal perception of mental health conditions in Ghana.

4.2.2 Religious Conceptions of Illness and Care

Ghana is a middle-income country with a population of more than 32 million, characterised by deep religious zeal (cf. Badu et al., 2018; Worldometer, 2022). Religion is an important regulator of social life as Ghanaians have a deep-seated tradition of religious observance, with three prominent belief groups, namely Christians (68.8%), Muslims (15.9%), and Animists (8.5%). Since religion is so entrenched in the lives of Ghanaians, the supranatural realm often plays a prominent role in explaining matters that are beyond comprehension for the average Ghanaian. Mental health challenges fall squarely into this category (Fournier, 2012), and most Ghanaians associate mental health issues with supranatural causes, such as witchcraft and (familial) curses (Ofori-Atta et al., 2010), while people suffering from mental health conditions are viewed with fear and suspicion as they are generally considered to be possessed by spirits (cf. Adu-Gyamfi, 2017; Fournier, 2012).

These beliefs cut across all societal classes. An interlocutor with over two decades of experience in mental health care in Ghana expressed astonishment at the number of highly educated Ghanaians who hold the belief that mental disorders have supranatural or spiritual causes.[7] The predominant perception that supranatural forces, evil spirits, curses, and bewitchment cause mental disorders (Adu et al., 2021; Adu-Gyamfi, 2017), reportedly exposes persons with mental illness to shunning and exclusion, as they are labelled witches or considered to be possessed by the devil. Dealing with mental health issues in Ghana can thus be a lonely experience as patients and carers are ignored by others, and at times even receive threats from their surroundings.[8] Stigmatisation prevents people from seeking help when they suffer from mental illness, as they are considered outcasts.[9] "If the person is a woman [with mental disorder], it will be difficult for her to find a husband. If it is a man, he will find it hard to find a wife, but also a job."[10]

As a result of Ghanaian societal attitudes towards people with mental health issues, there is a tendency to avoid getting a diagnosis based on standardised protocols, such as the DSM-5, for fear of the "courtesy stigma" (Goffman, 2009/1963) or stigma by association. Instead, an interlocutor, a psychologist with a life-long career in the Ghanaian mental health sector, notes that relatives tend to personalise the mental health issues. She points out that in her interactions with families of those suffering from mental health issues, these relatives ask whether they have done something wrong. "Instead of seeing it [mental illness] as a problem that can be solved. They personalise it as if they have failed."[11] In her view, this approach is what leads families to expose relatives suffering from

[7] Interview with Dr. B-O., Accra, Ghana (July 2017).

[8] Interview with Dr. C., Sakumono, Accra, Ghana. (May 2017).

[9] Interview with Dr. N., Accra Mall, Accra, Ghana (August 2017).

[10] Interview with Dr. N., Accra Mall, Accra, Ghana (August 2017).

[11] Interview with Dr. B-O, Accra, Ghana (July 2017).

mental disorders to abuse, neglect, and abandonment on the streets (Adu-Gyamfi, 2017). Once people personalise the mental illness of their family members, she noted, they cease to reason rationally, and hence can expose themselves and their loved ones to harm.

Combined, these factors and conditions drive those suffering mental disorders, along with their families, to seek answers in the divine realm. Because mental health challenges are seen to have spiritual origins, families' first call for help is often a religious institution, such as the church or prayer camp, and at times the pursuit of exorcisms by priests and spiritualists. The quest for divine intervention ties in divination, which is predicated on the notion that higher entities exist and that diviners have extraordinary capacities to communicate with those knowing entities (Beisel et al., 2018). However, the belief in higher entities and their abilities to offer relief to people with mental health challenges and their families, has reportedly led to instances of abuse by spiritualists who purport to heal mental disorders at prayer camps, shrines, and churches, where the mentally ill persons are chained or incarcerated (cf. Ofori-Atta et al., 2010; Read, 2019). Usually, these abuses go unquestioned or unpunished due to the desperation of those suffering from mental health issues, and of their families.

Negative perceptions of mental health in Ghana are further strengthened by mental health professionals who, like the average Ghanaian, at times hold the belief that there is a possibility that mental disorder has a spiritual causation (Read, 2019). This belief results in some of these health providers supporting approaches such as divine healing and prayer camps. These professionals thus do not see much contradiction in addressing mental health challenges through biomedical as well as spiritual means (cf. Read, 2019), but rather firmly believe in both approaches. Although we could argue that a pluralistic approach to tackling mental disorders is commendable, in Ghana this is problematic because people's belief in the supranatural causes of mental health issues has exposed patients to harm (Ofori-Atta et al., 2010; cf. Read, 2019). Psychologists discussing the trajectory of people who seek their help point to another serious implication. One interlocutor notes that "about 99% of the people who come here [to the practice] have had some sort of spiritual experience. They have been to see priests, spiritualists, shrines, and the like."[12] Another

[12] Interview with Dr. B-O., Accra, Ghana (July 2017).

interlocutor sharing experiences in his practice stated that patients "tell me that they've been to pastors, witchdoctors, traditional healers, but nothing seems to help them. Then someone tells them to go to the hospital; they might find redemption at the hospital."[13] However, "[b]y the time the people get here [that is to psychiatric hospital or psychological help] it has become worse. If it is a panic attack, by the time they get here it is a panic disorder. Which is more difficult to treat."[14] Another interlocutor adds that "by the time they come to the hospital, sometimes [it is too late]. It will shock you to know that even health workers do that. I know a doctor whose child had attention deficit. But by the time he sought help, it was almost too late."[15]

4.2.3 Stigmatisation and Mental Health Misinformation

Due to its association with the supranatural realm, many Ghanaians avoid mental health as a topic altogether. That means that they do not invest time in understanding the phenomenon. In its place, perceptions about mental health are informed by gossip about mental health patients and their families as being cursed or as having done something wrong. As a result of their limited knowledge of the phenomenon, most Ghanaians do not know the difference between mental health conditions such as depression and psychosis, while the psychologist is simply seen as a person who treats "mad people."[16] Therefore, when it comes to mental health in Ghana, perceptions are either black or white, with no differentiation of actual symptoms and diagnoses.[17]

Misconceptions are prevalent also in the more educated part of Ghanaian society, where there is a common perception that mental health is caused by faulty genes, and thus that mental disorders have a genetic foundation.[18] Traditionally, for instance, in most communities, before one marries into a house, the families do a search to ascertain whether there are genetic diseases in that house, including a history of mental

[13] Interview with Dr. W., 37 Military Hospital, Accra, Ghana (November 2017).

[14] Interview with Dr. C., Sakumono, Accra, Ghana (May 2017).

[15] Interview with Dr. B-O., Accra, Ghana (July 2017).

[16] Interview with Dr. N., Accra Mall, Accra, Ghana (August 2017).

[17] Interview with Dr. O-A., Korle-Bu, Accra (October 2017).

[18] Interview with Dr. O-A., Korle-Bu, Accra (October 2017).

illnesses. If mental illness is discovered in the family one wants to marry into, couples are discouraged from marrying each other.[19] However, increasingly in the higher educated Ghanaian circles, it is acknowledged that societal pressures, such as educational demands, career expectations, or loss of a loved one, are also sources of depression, anxiety, and other mental problems.[20] Another common perception is that mental illness is caused by poverty, which is preventing one from achieving one's goals in life. Other associations are made with failed love affairs or botched relationships, which could result in mental health problems. Expressions about mental health such as "*abo afa ni trim,*" which literally translates as "it has exploded in his/her head," support this, connoting that the person in question experiences mental health challenges as a result of a disappointment in life. Put differently, in the more educated quarters of Ghanaian society, there is increasingly knowledge that mental health could have multiple causes, including societal pressures or failed love encounters. Yet, despite the acknowledgement that societal pressures could be a source of mental health issues, the phenomenon remains broadly unknown, which is a major contributor to negative perceptions and stigmatisation of mental disorders in Ghana (Kleintjes et al., 2010).

Another issue that contributes to the negative societal association of mental health is that most Ghanaians have no idea what a psychologist does. According to a psychologist at a major hospital in Accra, "people think that psychologists read people's minds. They fear that you are going to know everything about them, including their fantasies and secrets. People fear that you are going to manipulate them." The limited knowledge people have about the job of mental health professionals tends to make members of the general public suspicious towards the providers. Mental health professionals must also regularly deal with prejudices. A Ghanaian psychologist who has been practicing since 1995 notes that "many people still believe that mental health is contagious."[21] This professional has had many moments in which people have avoided contact with her because they feared that since she deals with mental disorders, she might infect them with mental illness. Another psychologist has also had similar experiences with people shunning him in public:

[19] Interview with Dr. O-A., Korle-Bu, Accra (October 2017).

[20] Interview with Dr. O-A., Korle-Bu, Accra (October 2017).

[21] Interview with Dr. O-A., Korle-Bu, Accra Ghana. (October 2017).

"When I go to church, some people avoid sitting next to me because they believe that because I work with people with mental health issues, I might be carrying a virus or something that I could pass on to them, if they would sit next to me. Some people say to us that we look like our patients; dazed and confused, while others question how we can work with mad people."[22] Mental health thus carries a strong stigma in Ghana, not only towards patients, but also towards other people and professionals through association or "courtesy stigma" (Goffman, 2009/1963). The source of these misunderstandings, according to my interlocutors, is the limited understanding Ghanaians have of mental disorders and mental health professionals.

Mental health stigma is not only attached to sufferers and care providers, but also to psychological institutions. An interlocutor notes that "recognised national institutions have that stigma attached to them, for example, Accra Psychiatric Hospital."[23] As a result, another mental health practitioner points out that it "takes a big courage for the family to send the person [sufferer] to the psychiatric hospitals. If you are seen entering such a place, people start talking about you. There must be something wrong."[24] This has obvious implications for mental health care provision.

4.3 Standardisation and Mental Health Advocacy

Exposure to training, both in Ghana and abroad, has impacted how Ghanaian mental health professionals interrogate societal perceptions of mental health in their country, leading them to take action to try and inspire change. Standardisation or standardised protocols (Lampland & Star, 2009), such as DSM-5, are designed to facilitate other tasks (Beisel et al., 2018). In mental health-affiliated fields, standardisation facilitates the assessment, diagnosis, and treatment of mental health conditions. It is reminiscent[25] of testing as a critical means to help direct action (Beisel et al., 2018). Put differently, the standardised protocols, like diagnostic

[22] Interview with Dr. W., 37 Military Hospital, Accra, Ghana (November 2017).

[23] Interview with Dr. C., Sakumono, Accra, Ghana (May 2017).

[24] Interview with Dr. B-O., Accra, Ghana (July 2017).

[25] Interview with Dr. C., Sakumono, Accra, Ghana (May 2017).

tests, enable the professional to examine, discover, and prescribe the next line of action to help the patient. These protocols can in other words be considered devices to make the world predictable or reality more manageable (Calkins, 2016).

Generally, standardised protocols in clinical care are enforced by State institutions. In Ghana's mental health system, this is the responsibility of the Ghana Health Service's Mental Health Department,[26] with the support of professional bodies such as the Ghana Psychological Council, which issues licenses and certificates to mental health providers and practitioners. Standards exert a generative force as they stabilise and lock in categories about the world (Bowker & Star, 2000). As noted in the other chapters in this volume, in the (post)colonial Ghanaian context, biomedicine has a hegemonic position of perceived efficacy and modernity, compared to traditional and faith-based healing approaches to mental health (Kong et al., 2021; Kwame, 2021). Thus, despite the fact that the adoption of clinical mental health care so far remains limited in Ghana,[27] the global reach of international standardised protocols, such as the DSM-5, is important as it (gradually) increases trust in biomedical approaches to mental health, and by extension the work of mental health professionals' clinical assessment, diagnosis, and treatment.

This trend towards standardisation does not mean that standards ever completely overwrite Ghanaian cultural approaches to mental health and healing. As Lampland and Star (2009) note, standards are inherently localised, as they touch very specific communities. They thus always require distinct translations. According to an interlocutor in my study, professionals observe a duality in approach. Ghanaians alternate between traditional and biomedical interventions; in some cases, they embrace both approaches congruently. "We work with the different differentials and assessments. After that you are sure of what is going on and then you can start with the required treatment or therapy. So, more and more people are turning away from seeking strictly spiritual intervention and turning more and more to psychology for relief." From the Ghanaian

[26] Tasks of the Mental Health Department; https://ghs.gov.gh/mental-health-department/.

[27] It is estimated that traditional and faith-based systems are used exclusively by approximately 80% of people requiring mental health support on the African continent, and mental health professionals also emphasise the importance of cultural dynamics, such as the role of the church (WHO, 2019).

cultural perspective, this dual approach to seek relief is a safer choice, considering the stakes involved when it comes to mental health and the stigma associated with it.

Both locally and foreign-trained mental health professionals are tapping into this momentum to advocate further for the elimination of persistent stigma, and to alter perceptions of mental disorders and the mental health profession. As stated in the preceding paragraphs, mental health in Ghana is the backbencher of the medical profession in Ghana due to the country's focus on physical health. While mental health professionals are the lowest-paid specialists in Ghana's medical sector,[28] they also deal with societal prejudices and professional courtesy stigma (Goffman, 2009/1963). My interlocutors are frustrated due to the lack of appreciation for their difficult job of working in a society that does not value their skills and expertise, and which judges them for treating patients with mental disorders. That is why they want to change societal perceptions about mental health, while educating people in their society and advocating for those who suffer from mental health challenges. In the remainder of the chapter, the focus will be on the use of standardised international methods of diagnosis and assessment of mental disorders, such as the DSM-5, in advocacy and education activities undertaken by Ghanaian mental health professionals.

Standards and protocols in mental health play an important role in the advocacy efforts of Ghanaian mental health providers. A key function is in communicating the nature and differentiations of mental health. Professionals use categories of mental health laid down in the standard protocols of the DSM-5 to explain mental health symptoms to the public in concrete terms.

> When I make a presentation to organisations, institutions, the first thing I tell them is: 'I have some mental health issues'. (...) So that they know that mental health isn't just madness. I tell them that if I have a problem sleeping, that is a mental health issue. So I let people know that mental health doesn't necessarily mean you are going mad, you know. Then I tell them exactly what schizophrenia is, or what depression with psychotic features is ... I tell them that this is not madness. I explain the differences, that is how we do it.

[28] Interview with Dr. W., 37 Military Hospital, Accra, Ghana (November 2017).

If standardisation is aimed at validating knowledge through the logic of testing and diagnostics (Beisel et al., 2018), Ghanaian mental health professionals who seek to alter societal conceptions hope to mobilise a higher order of validity when sharing clinically defined understandings of mental health symptoms, and explaining the different disorders to lay people. Through this approach, the mental health providers try to convince their audience that mental health is a medical condition rather than a spiritual affair. By drawing on the DSM-5 and providing everyday examples, like insomnia and anxiety, the professionals seek to bring issues of mental health closer to people, with the goal of altering perceptions on mental health in Ghana.

My interlocutors believe they are making a difference through the use of the DSM-5 in their effort to expand mental health awareness. "We must tell people across society that mental health problems are really medical conditions that can be treated."[29] The goal of formulating the message in this manner is to reduce the stigma associated with mental health, while presenting mental health issues as medical conditions based on internationally agreed criteria. In particular, my interlocutors point to the importance of language and the value of standard terms. "When we engage with people, we try to use language that does not scare them. We try to explain to people what mental health entails in plain and clear language. We also say that it is a medical problem, not a spiritual one."[30] Since mental health issues scare Ghanaians due to their limited understanding of the phenomenon, the professionals aim to demystify mental health by breaking it down in clear and understandable terms, while emphasising that it is a medical condition which has nothing to do with witchcraft or demons. Standardisation in mental health is helping practitioners to demystify mental health as an evidence-based best practice which is founded on scientific rigour (Nortje et al., 2016).

The demystification, my interlocutors assert, "takes mental health away from the spiritual [realm]"[31] and reaffirms mental health disorders as actual medical conditions that can be treated. In their view, the use of international standardised terminology helps not only professionals, but also patients and their family explain that the mental health disorder is a

[29] Interview with Dr. B-O., Accra, Ghana (July 2017).

[30] Interview with Dr. N., Accra Mall, Accra, Ghana (August 2017).

[31] Interview with Dr. O-A., Korle-Bu, Accra Ghana (October 2017).

medical problem. Using these assessment tools and methods also makes it easier for people to seek help earlier. "Too often, people come to us too late because they don't know that we can assess them objectively and tell them exactly what they are going through or what they are suffering from."[32] If people can be helped quicker, and avoid exacerbating their condition due to delayed care, therapy, and medication, eventually societal perceptions of mental illness can improve, too.

As mental health professionals mobilise DSM-5 in their drive to educate the Ghanaian public about mental health, they are actively adapting their strategies to the Ghanaian context. Specifically, Ghanaian mental health professionals target spiritual leaders (priests, pastors) in their advocacy activities. As stated above, these religious leaders have a large following in Ghana. In the eyes of the professionals, the more knowledge these leaders are fed, the more people could potentially be reached. The mental health professionals claim to already see the impact of their efforts. For instance, although culturally, discussing issues around suicide is viewed with suspicion and scepticism in the Ghanaian cultural context (Eshun, 2003; Nukunya, 2003), my interlocutors report receiving invitations from renowned pastors to discuss this charged topic.[33] The mental health providers are also invited to talk about depression. Despite the complicated relations Ghanaians have with mental health in general and with these issues in particular, the location of advocacy in familiar contexts such as churches has allowed the advocates to bring knowledge about mental health closer to the society.

In addition, advocacy activities take place in a variety of other physical venues, such as schools and hospitals across the country, as well as in debates on health and mental health in Ghanaian mass media outlets. "Some of the media houses now have programs dealing with mental health so we join them."[34] My interlocutors report that there is not only growing knowledge about mental health in their country, but also a lot of demand from schools to engage with people on the topic. Until recently, mental health was not included in the curriculum at most schools across the country except for a few private schools with an international orientation. According to an interlocutor who has been working in the Ghanaian

[32] Interview with Dr. C., Sakumono, Accra, Ghana (May 2017).

[33] Interview with Dr. C., Sakumono, Accra, Ghana (May 2017).

[34] Interview with Dr. S., Accra Central, Ghana (August 2017).

education and mental health sectors for over a decade, "our people are not psychology savvy. They are not familiar with psychological terminologies so any time they hear things like depression or schizophrenia, they think: 'Am I crazy? Did I do something wrong? Is there something wrong with me?'"[35] For mental health professionals engaged in advocacy, knowledge, and awareness of mental health are thus crucial in changing perceptions. Through public education, Addy et al. (2021) note, mental health education can be introduced from the primary through to the university levels as a non-examinable subject taught by trained professionals with academic qualifications in, among other disciplines, psychology, psychiatry, and counselling. The scope of the mental health education could also cover common mental health problems, including the signs, symptoms, and triggers of mental health disorders, but also preventive measures, coping strategies, and support services (Addy et al., 2021). Advocates argue that such a program would improve knowledge about mental health in the country and mental health terminologies, and by extension alter perceptions of the phenomenon.

These examples provide additional evidence for the careful translation of standardised clinical knowledge into Ghanaian advocacy contexts. Advocacy and awareness-raising on mental health issues fall on the fruitful ground of Ghanaians cultural practices around counselling, which not least fits into a larger trend in Africa, related to the emergence of the middle class and to experiences with HIV/AIDS counselling (Bröer et al., 2016; Vaugh, 2016). Culturally, "Ghanaians have always believed in counselling; they love it! In church, every person sees themselves as a counsellor. It is all about advice; telling you what to do and what not to do."[36] What the psychologist seems to imply here is that Ghanaians' readiness to routinely give and receive advice on various matters ranging from employment and education to marital issues is an entry point to mental health advocacy. These practices provide people relief from challenges without them having to resort to professional therapists. Here, help seekers and informal counsellors interact with each other in a non-professional manner or setting to arrive at some sort of resolution for whatever problems they are facing. Another respondent corroborates this view and adds: "I compare counselling to going for confession [like

[35] Interview with Y. A., Ring Road, Accra, Ghana (October 2017).

[36] Interview with Dr. B-O., Accra, Ghana (July 2017).

Catholics do]. You share whatever issues or challenges you are facing with the therapist. Ghanaians consulting or seeing their pastors with their problems, they are engaging in some form of counselling."[37]

Counselling as a kind of informal advice platform provides a low-stakes context where ideas are exchanged, which in turn leads to a form of relief, but also the opportunity to change perceptions. This approach draws from different worldviews and disciplines to arrive at a way of doing things that fits into the Ghanaian understanding of mental health, counselling, and treatments. It shows that despite pervasive negative conceptions of mental health, there are avenues for changing such perceptions that are socially and culturally rooted in Ghanaian society and traditions.

4.4 Conclusion

Medical anthropology helps us understand how competing conceptions of mental health come together in specific contexts in Ghana; here specifically, in treatment and advocacy activities, and in how standard diagnostics impact conceptions of mental health in these domains. Medical anthropology brings local and global knowledge together, while the Ghanaian mental health providers mediate cultural dynamics and belief systems in relation to clinical treatment and the standard international protocols in their care practices.

The level of education of Ghanaians has been on the rise since independence, in tandem with that of mental health professionals. The consequence of this is that increasingly "people understand social and global views,"[38] including standard clinical perceptions around mental health. The growing knowledge contributes to changing understandings of mental health challenges, while helping to reach wider quarters of society through its order of validity. At the same time, standards are necessarily localised. "Ghanaian churches are learning about mental health and pastors are taking courses to enable them to counsel their congregations. They also want to learn to better distinguish between what is strictly in the spiritual realm and what is beyond them. That is, what is for the psychologist or psychiatrist."[39] As a result of this growing

[37] Interview with Dr. N., Accra Mall, Accra, Ghana (August 2017).

[38] Interview with Dr. O-A., Korle-Bu, Accra Ghana (October 2017).

[39] Interview with Dr. C., Sakumono, Accra, Ghana (May 2017).

knowledge, psychologists are seeing that "more and more Ghanaians are realising that behind the spiritual, there could also be something psychological." This, the mental health professional adds, has real-life impacts. "A lot of ordinary people are coming to me now. I work on strictly appointments basis. I can tell you I have a full agenda!"[40] Specifically, Ghanaian mental health professionals observe that their awareness campaigns have resulted—although it is an unintended consequence—in more people calling on their services, indicating the growing knowledge and patronising of mental health services.

Despite the positive developments and changing tide in relation to the perceptions of mental health in Ghana, there is still a long way to go. An interlocutor formulated it in the following manner: "It still doesn't occur to some Ghanaian doctors that they should refer people to the psychologist. Once, at a meeting of medical specialists where we were discussing the case of a patient, I had to raise my hand to point out that psychological guidance should be part of the patient's recovery and treatment plan."[41] Changing perceptions in a society like Ghana is a gradual process that will take more time. Despite the evolution in perception of mental health in Ghana, even among certain medical professionals, the recognition of the necessity of including mental health in patients' recovery has still to sink in.

Although officially recognised State institutions use and implement DSM-5 standardised protocols for assessment, diagnosis, and treatment of mental health issues in Ghana, practitioners and patients who are associated with these hospitals still remain stigmatised. The status of these bodies as recognised institutions does not fully insulate them from negative societal perceptions and stigma. Stigmatisation therefore continues to drive sufferers and their families to go "underground"[42] to seek help from traditionalists and faith-based organisations. "Stigma can drive families into despair. That is why you find them going to all these people [pastors and traditional healers]. I don't know if it is a defence mechanism. They tell themselves that [someone is bewitching] their child, so they have to go for deliverance. And then they have a lot of pastors who

[40] Interview with Dr. C., Sakumono, Accra, Ghana (May 2017).

[41] Interview with Dr. N., Accra Mall, Accra, Ghana (August 2017).

[42] Interview with Dr. B-O., Accra, Ghana (July 2017).

also tell them that they can deliver their family member."[43] It appears that the fear of being stigmatised by society is far greater for some families than their fear of entrusting mental health sufferers to potential charlatans, instead of to a recognised institution that uses standard protocols to assess, diagnose, and treat mental health issues.

In this perception, although one would expect that the use of standardised protocols such as the DSM-5 to assess, diagnose and treat mental health issues would provide a trustworthy foundation to get mental health care in Ghana, it appears that in the Ghanaian case, societal perceptions and stigma remain more powerful. The material presented here points towards the conclusion that people who have been medically diagnosed may suffer even more stigma, not only due to the disease, but also because of their affiliation or relationship to a recognised mental health institution which may also be stigmatised. The use of standardised protocols in clinical care hence does not automatically reduce the level of stigma associated with mental health in Ghana. Instead, awareness and advocacy are more complex and lengthy processes. Yet, standardisation in Ghana's mental health system can contribute to awareness-building about mental health as a medical condition rather than a curse, especially when working hand in hand with intermediary institutions such as the churches and other counselling practices. These manifestations of mental health experts' advocacy efforts are an important component in the bid to thaw the frosty relationship between the Ghanaian general public and mental health. That there is still a long way to go in changing perceptions of mental health in Ghana, is not least also due to the continued lack of investment in the mental health infrastructure in the country and the lack of financial resources from the State's budget. Without adequate clinical infrastructure, raising awareness can only lead us so far.

References

Addy, N. D., Agbozo, F., Runge-Ranzinger, S., & Grys, P. (2021). Mental health difficulties, coping mechanisms and support systems among school-going adolescents in Ghana: A mixed-methods study. *PLoS ONE, 16*(4), e0250424.

Adika, D. M., Chutiyami, M., Dathini, H., Adamu, H., & Chutiyami, M. (2017). Maternal mortality in Ghana: An exploration of partners' perception about

[43] Interview with Dr. B-O., Accra, Ghana (July 2017).

factors that contributed to their wife's death. *Int J Community Med Public Health, 4*(11), 4018–4024.

Adomakoh, C. C. (1972a). Mental health patients: A castle road profile. *Ghana Medical Journal, 2*(1), 65–71.

Adomakoh, C. C. (1972b). Prevalence of motor disorders in Phenothiazine treated psychotics in mental hospital. *Ghana Medical Journal, 2*(1), 149–153.

Adu, P., Jurcik, T., & Grigoryev, D. (2021). Mental health literacy in Ghana: Implications for religiosity, education and stigmatization. *Transcultural Psychiatry, 58*(4), 516–531.

Adu-Gyamfi, S. (2017). Mental health service in Ghana: A review of the case. *International Journal of Public Health Science, 6*(4), 299–313.

Affinnih, Y. H. (2005). Pilot study of the relationship between drug misuse and violence among drug addicts in Greater Accra, Ghana: The south of Saharan Africa case. *Substance Use & Misuse, 40*(6), 813–822.

Anum, A., Washington-Nortey, M., & Dzokoto, V. (2020). Strategic planning in LAMIC mental health research: A Ghana case study. *International Journal of Mental Health, 49*(2), 128–156.

Arias, D., Taylor, l, Ofori-Atta, A., & Bradley, E. H. (2016). Prayer camps and biomedical care in Ghana: Is collaboration in mental health care possible? *PLoS One, 11*(9), e0162305.

Asare, J. B. (2001). Mental health in Ghana. *Ghana Medical Journal, 35*(3), 105–120.

Awenva, A. D., Read, U. M., Ofori-Attah, A. L., Doku, V. C., Akpalu, B., Osei, A. O., & Flisher, A. J. (2010). From mental health policy development in Ghana to implementation: What are the barriers? *African Journal of Psychiatry, 13*, 184–191.

Badu, E., O'Brien, A. P., & Mitchell, R. (2018). An integrative review of potential enablers and barriers to accessing mental health services in Ghana. *Health Research Policy and Systems, 16*, 1–19.

Beisel, U., Calkins, S., & Rottenburg, R. (2018). Divining, testing, and the problem of accountability. *HAU: Journal of Ethnographic Theory, 8*(1–2), 109–113.

Bowker, G.C., & Star, S.L. (2000). *Sorting things out: Classification and its consequences*. MIT Press.

Bröer, C., Spronk, R., & Kraak, V. (2016). Exploring the ADHD Diagnosis in Ghana: Between disrespect and lack of institutionalization. In M. Bergey, A. Filipe, P. Conrad, & I. Singh (Eds.), *Global perspectives on ADHD: Social dimensions of diagnosis and treatment in 16 countries* (pp. 354–375). Johns Hopkins University Press.

Calkins, S. (2016). *Who knows tomorrow? Uncertainty in north-eastern Sudan*. Berghahn.

Canavan, M., Sipsma, H., Jack, H., Ohene, S., Rohrbaugh, R., Bradley, E., Ofori-Atta, A., & MHaPP Research Consortium. (2016). Psychoactive prescription practices for serious mental and neurological illness in Ghana: Data from the mental health and poverty project (MHaPP). *International Journal of Mental Health, 45*(4), 223–235.

Doku, V. C. K., Wusu-Takyi, A., & Awakame, J. (2012). Implementing the mental health act in Ghana: Any challenges ahead? *Ghana Medical Journal, 46*(4), 241–250.

Eshun, S. (2000). Role of gender and rumination in suicide ideation: A comparison of college samples from Ghana and the United States. *Cross-Cultural Research, 34*(3), 250–263.

Eshun, S. (2003). Sociocultural determinants of suicide ideation: A comparison between American and Ghanaian college samples. *Suicide and Life Threatening Behaviour, 33*(2), 165–171.

Eshun, S., Chang, E. C., & Owusu, V. (1998). Cultural and gender differences in responses to depressive mood: A study of college students in Ghana and the USA. *Personality and Individual Differences, 24*(4), 581–583.

Field, M. J. (1958). Mental disorder in rural Ghana. *The Journal of Mental Science, 104*(437), 1043–1051.

Field, M. J. (1960). *Search for security: An ethno psychiatric study of rural Ghana*. Faber and Faber.

Foster, J. B., & Ingram, T. T. S. (1962). Familial cerebro-macular degeneration and ataxia. *Journal of Neurology, Neurosurgery, and Psychiatry, 25*(1), 63–68.

Fournier, O. A. (2012). The status of mental health care in Ghana, West Africa and signs of progress in the greater Accra region. *Berkeley Undergraduate Journal, 24*(3). https://doi.org/10.5070/B3243007890

Goffman, E. (2009/1963). *Stigma: Notes on the management of spoiled identity*. Simon & Schutser.

Government of Ghana. (2012). *Ghana: Act No. 846 of 2012, Mental Health Act*. National Legislative Bodies/National Authorities.

Hjelmeland, H., Akotia, C. S., Owens, V., Knizek, B. L., Nordvik, H., & Schroeder, R. (2008). Self-reported suicidal behavior and attitudes toward suicide and suicide prevention among psychology students in Ghana, Uganda, and Norway. *Crisis, 29*(1), 20–31.

Kleintjes, S., Lund, C., & Flisher, A. J. (2010). A situational analysis of child and adolescent mental health services in Ghana, Uganda, South Africa and Zambia. *African Journal of Psychiatry, 13*(2), 132–139.

Kong, C., Campbell, M., Kpobi, L., Swartz, L., & Atuire, C. (2021). The hermeneutics of recovery: Facilitating dialogue between African and Western mental health frameworks. *Transcultural Psychiatry, 60*(3), 428–442.

Kpobi, L., Read, U. M., Selormey, R. K., & Colucci, E. (2023). 'We are all working toward one goal. We want people to become well': A visual exploration of what promotes successful collaboration between community mental health workers and healers in Ghana. *Transcultural Psychiatry, 61*(1), 30–46.

Kwame, A. (2021). Integrating traditional medicine and healing into the Ghanaian mainstream health system: Voices from within. *Qualitative Health Research, 31*(10), 1847–1860.

Lampland, M., & Star, S. L. (2009). *Standards and their stories: How quantifying, classifying, and formalizing practices shape everyday life*. Cornell University Press.

Lauterbach, K. (2010). Becoming a pastor youth and aspirations in Ghana. *Young, 18*(3), 259–278.

Meyer, B. (2012). Religious and secular, 'spiritual' and 'physical' in Ghana. What Matters? In C. Bender & A. Taves (Eds.), *Ethnographies of value in a (not so) secular age* (pp. 86–118). Columbia University Press.

Mhlanga, S. S. G. (2023). *The philosophy of integrating medical anthropology & clinical psychology: Mental health & soul health*. WestBow Press.

Nortje, G., Oladeji, B., Gureje, O., & Seedat, S. (2016). Effectiveness of traditional healers in treating mental disorders: A systematic review. *The Lancet Psychiatry, 3*(2), 154–170.

Nukunya, G. K. (2003). *Tradition and change in Ghana*. Ghana University Press.

Ofori-Atta, A., Read, U. M., & Lund, C. (2010). A situation analysis of mental health services and legislation in Ghana: Challenges for transformation. *African Journal of Psychiatry, 13*(2), 99–108.

Omar, M. A., Green, A. T., Bird, P. K., Mirzoev, T., Flisher, A. J., Kigozi, F., Lund, C., Mwanza, J., & Ofori-Atta, A. L. (2010). Mental health policy process: A comparative study of Ghana, South Africa, Uganda and Zambia. *International Journal of Mental Health Systems, 4*, 24. https://doi.org/10.1186/1752-4458-4-24

Osei, A., Roberts, M., & Crabbe, J. (2011). The new Ghana mental health bill. *International Psychiatry, 8*(1), 8–9.

Rathod, S., Pinninti, N., Irfan, M., Gorczynski, P., Rathod, P., Gega, L., & Naeem, F. (2017). Mental health service provision in low-and middle-income countries. *Health Services Insights, 10*. https://doi.org/10.1177/1178632917694350

Read, U. M. (2019). Rights as relationships: Collaborating with faith healers in community mental health in Ghana. *Culture, Medicine and Psychiatry, 43*, 613–635.

Read, U. M., & Doku, V. C. K. (2012). Mental health research in Ghana: A literature review. *Ghana Medical Journal, 46*(2), 29–38.

Turkson, S. N., & Dua, A. N. (1996). A study of the social and clinical characteristics of depressive illness among Ghanaian women (1988–1992). *West African Journal of Medicine, 15*(2), 85–90.

Turkson, S. N. (2000). Schizophrenia—The spirit possessed 23 year old male from rural Kpando Dzoanti, Volta region in Ghana: Case report. *East African Medical Journal, 77*(11), 629–630.

Vaugh, M. (2016). Changing the subject? Psychological counseling in eastern Africa. *Public Culture, 28*(3), 499–517.

Walker, G. H., & Osei, A. (2017). Mental health law in Ghana. *Bjpsych International, 14*(2), 38–39.

Walters, V., Avotri, J. Y., & Charles, N. (1999). "Your heart is never free": Women in Wales and Ghana talking about distress. *Canadian Psychology/psychologie Canadienne, 40*(2), 129–142.

World Health Organization. (2019). WHO global report on traditional and complementary medicine 2019. Retrieved March 6, 2024, from https://www.who.int/publications/i/item/978924151536

Worldometer. (2022). https://www.worldometers.info/

CHAPTER 5

Traditional Medicine in Ghana: Statistical Production and Professionalisation of Practitioners, Practice, and Products

Diana Amoni Ntewusu

5.1 Introduction

In 2019, I started fieldwork on traditional medicine practice in Ghana for my doctoral thesis. This research took me to the office of the Secretary of the Greater Accra chapter of the Ghana National Association of Traditional Healers. The visit allowed me to attend the Association's general monthly meeting, and to observe the extent to which statistical concerns were paramount in the practice of traditional medicine in Ghana. Records were kept on how many members were duly registered as qualified practitioners with the Traditional Medicine Practice Council (TMPC). The

I did not receive any funding to do this work. Therefore I have no conflict of interest.

D. A. Ntewusu (✉)
Science and Technology Policy Research Institute, Council for Scientific and Industrial Research (CSIR—STEPRI), Accra, Ghana
e-mail: dantewusu@csir-stepri.org

A. Thiel and S. A. Ntewusu (eds.), *The Social Life of Health Data*,
https://doi.org/10.1007/978-981-97-3500-6_5

Council has the mandate and authority, provided under the Traditional Medicine Practice Act of 2000 (Act 575), to register and regulate the activities of all traditional medicine practitioners and their practices.

Individual practitioners are supposed to demonstrate membership in an association of practitioners for the purposes of easy identification, registration, and licensing. According to Act 575, the Council shall determine and enforce a code of ethics for traditional medicine practice in conjunction with an association of traditional medicine practitioners duly recognised by the Minister of Health. Furthermore, the question of how many members had their products registered and licensed by the Food and Drugs Authority (FDA) was of great importance to the Association. How many products, along with their indications, each member had registered was equally important. Therefore, members were admonished and encouraged to have their products registered by the FDA so as not to drag the name of the Association into disrepute.

The mandate of the FDA, under part seven of the Public Health Act (PHA) of 2012 (ACT 851), among others, is to regulate the production and sale of all food and drugs, including herbal medicine, in Ghana. Section 118 of the Act requires that all medicines, including herbal medicines, be registered, while section 130 of the Act ensures that the premises where these products are manufactured meet the minimum hygiene requirements for good manufacturing practices. Accordingly, no practitioner is allowed to prepare, manufacture, store, sell, or transport herbal medicine unless it is duly registered by the FDA (ACT 851, 2012). These regulations, in effect, address the problem of traditional medicine practitioners operating without the requisite authorisation and expertise, thereby endangering the lives of their clients (Chary & Sargent, 2016; Craig, 2011; Marsland, 2007; Mpinga et al., 2013).

This chapter sets out to explore the production of statistics on traditional medicine practitioners, their practices, and products in Ghana, and how these quantifications participate in the construction of professional bodies of herbal practitioners. Drawing on findings from qualitative interviews, archival sources, relevant data, and documents provided by the TMPC, FDA, and other stakeholders in the industry, the chapter provides a descriptive analysis of registered practitioners, and their practices and products. Of critical interest is the way practitioners respond to the various standardising forms and procedures emanating from regulatory practices, as well as to the purported imposition on them of professionalism, elements of which they view as running counter to the values of traditional healing.

The chapter will delve into key issues such as the number of practitioners registered by the TMPC, the various products registered by the FDA, along with their indications, and the gendered dynamics that the registers present. These discussions are preceded by a brief description of the developmental trajectory of the practice of traditional medicine in Ghana. The chapter concludes that there is no way one can understand traditional medical practice in Ghana without recourse to the statistics generated through regulatory standardising procedures, and without understanding the effects of these standards on practitioners, practices, and products.

5.2 The Developmental Trajectory of Traditional Medicine in Ghana

In Ghana, since independence, successive governments have made frantic efforts to satisfy the societal need for safe, efficient, and quality healthcare delivery across the nation. These efforts have mainly taken the form of formulating policies to support and regulate the practice of traditional medicine. Historically, attempts at controlling traditional medicine were initiated by colonial authorities under the guise of ridding the practice of quacks, superstition, and witchcraft activities (Adu-Gyamfi, 2015). Thus, as biomedicine gradually planted roots and gained dominance over traditional medicine in society, the Gold Coast became medically pluralistic by the close of the nineteenth century (Addae, 1996; Adu-Gyamfi, 2010; Osseo-Asare, 2016). The power, prestige, and wide utilisation enjoyed by biomedicine gave it structural superiority over traditional medicine over the years (Boateng et al., 2016).

As noted by Adu-Gyamfi (2015, p. 59), for the colonial authorities, traditional medicine was the "ignorance of the indigenous people couched in a belief in magic and witchcraft that cannot be explained by reason which resulted in a state of fear." Thus, traditional healers were denied official recognition by the colonialists. The struggle that ensued resulted in the healers getting together to form associations. The Society of African Herbalists was formed at Sekondi in 1931, with Kwesi Aaba as its president (Adu-Gyamfi, 2010; Osseo-Asare, 2016). Members, among other things, sought to raise the standard of the local practice of medicine, and to gain official recognition and the freedom to practice. At the time of British rule, the Native Physicians Control Bye-Laws governed traditional medical practice in the country. These laws resulted in several challenges in the development of traditional medicine and its practice. For example, in the 1940s the Secretary for Native Affairs had indicated his displeasure at the proliferation of traditional medicine practice facilities, and the pressure that healers put on the administration for official recognition. He stated, "I am not in favour of any bye-laws or licensing system which will imply official recognition and licensing authority that the licensee was a fit and proper person to practice medicine" (PRAAD Koforidua, ADM/KD 6/9/496).

When biomedicine was still in its embryonic state in the colony, the Secretary for Native Affairs considered it necessary to popularise it as opposed to traditional medicine. This was to avoid the possibility of people visiting traditional healers instead of the health facilities established by the colonial administration. The colonial administrators initially attributed ill health, especially issues of mental health or neurosis, to a state of imbalance arising out of poverty and illiteracy (see also Chapter 4, this volume). However, the healing provided in shrines, including "Brukum" and "Hwemisu," involving the use of plants, guaranteed some relief of sickness in body and mind (PRAAD Koforidua, ADM/KD 29/6/69). This, to some extent, made the colonial administrators reconsider their stance, even though not permanently, on the issue of ill health and medicine in the African's understanding. For "fetishes" were avenues through which people found healing without necessarily having recourse to witchcraft, something biomedicine could not accomplish satisfactorily (Twumasi, 2005). Regarding this point, Twumasi (2005, p. 168) rightly concluded thus:

> The limited utility of scientific medicine in the area of mental illness leaves open a relatively permanent area of chronic non-capacitating ills within which traditional medicine may survive and may continue in a complementary structural position, at least in the rural setting. This point is predicated on the idea that in the field of psychiatry, traditional medicine or its functional equivalent will continue to operate in this area.

Thus, to gain official recognition, some healers, working through the associations, sought to distance themselves from the cultural and traditional values attached to traditional healing and classified themselves simply as herbalists, as shown in the case of the Society of African Herbalists. This had serious implications for the developmental trajectory of traditional medicine in Ghana, because healers, through their segmented associations, continued to struggle amongst themselves over whose practice was authentic and traditional.

When Ghana finally gained independence in 1957, the first president, Dr. Kwame Nkrumah, showed tremendous interest in traditional medicine. Nkrumah's interest was influenced by pan-Africanist ideologies, which he well expressed on several platforms (Droney, 2014). For him, decolonisation was not only a political project, but also involved a change in mentality. Thus, at the inauguration of the Institute of African Studies at the University of Ghana in 1963, Nkrumah stated: (J. H. Kwabena Nketia Archive University of Ghana, Legon, IAS/3/1/44, Nkrumah Papers, Undated).

> We must regard education as the "gateway to the enchanted cities of the mind" and not only as a means to personal economic security and social privilege. Indeed, education consists not only in the sum of what a man knows, or the skill with which he can put this to his advantage. In my view, a man's education must also be measured in terms of the soundness of his judgement of people and things, and in his power to understand and appreciate the needs of his fellow men and to be of service to them. The educated man should be so sensitive to the conditions around him that he makes it his chief endeavour to improve those conditions for the good of all.[1]

With these ideas, he assigned the University of Science and Technology (UST), now Kwame Nkrumah University of Science and Technology (KNUST), to undertake extensive research into plant medicine (Memoir of Dr. Ampofo, undated). It is important to add that beyond the Pan-Africanist orientation of Nkrumah, his interest in traditional medicine was also due to a personal encounter with a female healer at Larteh, near Akropong, in the Eastern Region. Archival records indicate that Nana Ekua Oparebea, a traditional priestess at Larteh, treated Nkrumah for a chronic "head, chest, cough and sneeze with herbs" in 1961. The success of this treatment resulted in the State paying the healer two hundred

[1] J. H. Kwabena Nketia Archive University of Ghana, Legon, IAS/3/1/44, Nkrumah Papers, Undated.

British pounds at that time (PRAAD Accra, ADM 4/3/115, Report of Commission of Enquiry into the Kwame Nkrumah Properties, 1966). Nkrumah thus supported every move geared towards the development of indigenous medical knowledge systems to enhance healthcare delivery in the country. Dr. Nkrumah, Nana Akua Oparebea, and Mr. Mensah-Dapaa, a Research Fellow of the Academy of Arts and Sciences held discussions regarding the need to develop traditional medicine. Subsequently, on 7th April 1962, the Ghana Psychic and Traditional Healing Association (GPTHA) was inaugurated at Larteh by the then Minister of Health, Mr. A. E. Inkumsah (PRAAD Koforidua, ADM/KD/31/6/684).

Adu-Gyamfi (2015) notes that an association with the same name had sprung up in the 1950s for the same purpose. This earlier association metamorphosed into the GPTHA, which was inaugurated by Dr. Nkrumah in 1962. This group was different from the Society of African Herbalists in that it had presidential support. It was authorised to bring on board all expertise in traditional healing to meet the health needs of the Ghanaian populace. At the time, the GPTHA had the blessings of the president to "uphold, protect and promote the best in the traditions invested by the ancestors in the Indigenous Priest Healers including priestesses and herbalists in Ghana" (Adu-Gyamfi, 2015, p. 59).

Again, archival records reveal that there were attempts already in the 1960s to enhance and encourage the utilisation of traditional medicine throughout the country. In his address at Nsawam on the 16th of October 1963, Mr. E. H. T. Korboe, Regional Commissioner for Eastern Region stated as follows (PRAAD, Koforidua, ADM/KD/31/6/684):

> As we are all aware it is the ardent wish of Osagyefo the President that all avenues to protect and promote the health of the citizens of Ghana should be explored in order to build up healthy, strong, and able-bodied citizens both in mind and body and well fitted to play their part in the great special and economic reconstruction of the country. It is in keeping with this wish that this Association has been formed in order to tap and make available all the accredited talents and services in the age of traditional and cultural methods of healing diseases to the greater benefit of Ghana. Indeed, we are all aware that the system of healing diseases using herbs has been the practice of our forefathers since time immemorial.[2]

[2] PRAAD, Koforidua, ADM/KD/31/6/684.

After the overthrow of Kwame Nkrumah, however, subsequent governments did not follow through with the blueprint that had been established for the Association. Dr. Nkrumah had planned that the Association would collaborate with the Centre for Plant Medicine Research at Mampong-Akuapem to execute its mandate. In Dr. Ampofo's words (Dr. Ampofo's memoirs, Undated):

> The Centre was given a specific mandate. The first mandate was to conduct and promote scientific research relating to the improvement of plant medicine. Actually, for the real method of the research process, Dr Nkrumah formed the National Psychic and Traditional Healing Association which is all over the country. This association was meant to feed doctors of the Centre with information on traditional medicine.

However, some members of the Association eventually became an integral part of the Centre's activities in the promotion and utilisation of traditional medicine in Ghana when the Centre was finally established in the early 1970s. It bears mention that the name of the Association changed after Dr. Nkrumah was overthrown, from Ghana Psychic and Traditional Healing Association to Ghana Psychic and Traditional Healers' Association.

Meanwhile, the GPTHA became relevant when the Primary Health Care (PHC) programme was adopted and implemented in 1978, with its goal to provide health for all by the year 2000 (Anyinam, 1989). The Ministry of Health (MOH) recommended at that time that traditional healers, especially traditional birth attendants (TBAs), be involved in the development of health planning. Thus, through the activities of the GPTHA, traditional medical knowledge was harnessed for an improved PHC programme in the country. At the local level, the PHC depended on all categories of health practitioners, including traditional healers and birth attendants, who were available and qualified for the provision of health care. These traditional healthcare practitioners were trained together with the mainstream practitioners, to work as a team in response to the health needs of their respective communities, using local resources (Anyinam, 1989; Isola, 2013; Le Grand & Wondergem, 1990).

In 1985, a survey was conducted on the pharmaceutical landscape of Ghana with special reference to the capacity needs of traditional medicine production (Boateng et al., 2016). To ensure better coordination of activities in the traditional medicine landscape, a Traditional and Alternative

Medicine Unit was established under the MOH in 1991. This unit was elevated to a directorate in 2003 and is now known as the Traditional and Alternative Medicine Directorate (TAM-D). TAM-D superintends all activities within the traditional medicine industry, and is responsible for policy formulation under the auspices of the MOH.

In the meantime, new groups and associations of traditional health practitioners continued to emerge. Interestingly, traditional healers have had to continue to struggle for equal status with their biomedical counterparts, even though since independence the State had shown interest in developing traditional medicine, as indicated above. This struggle can be attributed to the colonial legacy of the superiority enjoyed by biomedicine over traditional medicine. Therefore, to bring traditional practitioners together, and to better understand and support their activities, the government facilitated the formation of a federation of the major traditional health practitioner associations. This gave birth to the Ghana Federation of Traditional Medicine Practitioners (GHAFTRAM) in 1999. Currently, GHAFTRAM is constituted of the Traditional Herbalist Association; Plant Medicine and Traditional Healers Association; Ghana Muslims Traditional Healers Association; Ghana Psychic and Traditional Healers Association; Ghana Association of Medical Herbalists; and Ghana National Association of Traditional Healers.

The Traditional Medicine Practice Act (TMPA) (Act 575) was enacted in the year 2000 to facilitate the establishment of the Traditional Medicine Practice Council (TMPC). As indicated already, TMPC is the regulator of the practice of traditional medicine, and is mandated to register all practitioners of traditional and alternative medicine in Ghana.

To further enhance the image of the practice of traditional medicine, the government established the Department of Herbal Medicine at the Faculty of Pharmacy, Kwame Nkrumah University of Science and Technology (KNUST) in the year 2000, to award the Bachelor of Science Degree in Herbal Medicine. The course is based on clinical and pharmaceutical aspects of herbal medicine, wherein one qualifies as a Medical Herbalist (MH) at the end of a four-year training programme. A recent development is the establishment of an Institute of Traditional and Alternative Medicine (ITAM) in September 2019 at the University of Health and Allied Sciences (UHAS). Since 2005, graduates from the Department of Herbal Medicine have taken over the professional and institutional practice of herbal medicine in Ghana.

Finally, in 2005, the government developed the Policy Guidelines on Traditional Medicine Development, which were aimed at providing a general policy direction or framework on which the government's short to long-term plans on traditional medicine would be based. A very central provision in the Policy Guidelines is the call to integrate traditional medicine into mainstream healthcare. Scholars have argued that the emergence of a wide range of healthcare needs has made it imperative for most post-colonial States to explore all forms of healing methods to maintain a healthy population (Harilal, 2009; Sujatha & Abraham, 2009). To be centralised and recognised, these forms of healing methods, including traditional medicine, must be regulated by the State. For this reason, State policies target traditional medicine through regulation, to give it the necessary recognition and bring it up to the required standard.

Since 2011, attempts have been made by the State to integrate traditional herbal medicine into mainstream healthcare on a pilot basis in 17 selected district hospitals across the country. However, it is reported that there is no available policy document outlining the goals and scope of integrating the practice into mainstream healthcare, leading to a varied understanding and level of acceptance by the stakeholders involved (Boateng et al., 2016). Consequently, the integration process has been slow, without much to show over the years. For example, Ampomah et al. (2023) indicate that even though the practice of integration is highly acceptable among traditional medicine practitioners and patients within the catchment area of the policy, its implementation is fraught with a myriad of barriers. Various factors have been acknowledged as barriers to implementation, including financial constraints in traditional medical practice, resulting in shortages of herbal products in the facilities; a failure by their biomedical counterparts within the implementing facilities to recognise and recommend traditional medicine practitioners; unbalanced professional training opportunities in favour of biomedical practitioners; a high rate of non-disclosure of previous use of herbal medicines to biomedical practitioners; and poor coordination and collaboration in patient care between biomedical practitioners and traditional medicine practitioners (Agyei-Baffour et al., 2017, Ampomah et al., 2023, Asante & Avornyo, 2013, Boateng et al., 2016). These findings reveal that Ghana still runs an essentially pluralistic medical system with parallel delivery models, in which all systems independently provide care within their legitimately defined mandates (Ampomah et al., 2023).

In the following section, I provide a descriptive analysis of the basic features of data available on the regulation of traditional medicine practitioners and their products.

5.3 The Politics of Standards and Professionalisation

Star and Lampland (2009) posit that to "standardize an action, process or thing, means, at some level, to screen out unlimited diversity." However, the resulting standards, which do not develop acontextually, often constitute or suggest ethics and values with great consequences for groups and individuals (Nyika, 2007, 2009; Star & Lampland, 2009). Notwithstanding, the political and social dynamics in the patronage and utilisation of traditional medicine in Ghana have centred mostly on issues of standardisation, based on biomedical scientific processes. This has been promoted because of the increasing emphasis on evidence-based practice in healthcare delivery across the globe (Feng et al., 2017; Nyika, 2009).

As the discussion above has shown, Ghana's traditional medicine standardisation agenda, which began before the country's independence in 1957, has come a long way, albeit slowly, due to inconsistencies and contestations from several positions—involving colonialists, the State, the biomedical fraternity, and traditional healers. The TMPA of 2000 (Act 575) and the PHA of 2012 (ACT 851), from which the TMPC and the FDA derive their respective mandates, have been the most effective (to some extent) standardising agents in recent times. These regulations spell out the role of a practitioner and the nature of their standardised practices and products. Act 575 defines "practitioner" as a traditional medicine practitioner whose practice uses herbs and any other natural products, and also adds that a person shall not operate or own premises as a practitioner, or produce herbal medicine for sale, unless that person is registered per the Act. Also, a "practice" is a traditional medicine practice and the "premises" for practice include a house, building, structure, tent, caravan, land, ship, boat, an aircraft, and a mechanically propelled vehicle (ACT 575).

Practitioners seeking to be registered, submit applications to the Registrar of the Council and approval is subject to the satisfaction of the Board that applicants have proficiency in the practice of traditional medicine. Also, the application should have been endorsed by any two of the following: the district chairman of the Association; the traditional ruler of the community; or the District Co-ordinating Director. Names of successful applicants are entered in the register of practitioners and they are issued with certificates of registration upon the payment of the prescribed fee, which currently stands at GHS 350 (approximately 35 USD). Certificates of registration are subject to yearly renewals, as they expire on the 31st of December each year. This law came into full force in September 2007.

Even though, in line with current global trends (Mpinga et al., 2013), Act 575 gives recognition to all forms of Traditional, Alternative and Complementary medical practices in the country, only practitioners of indigenous medicine are considered in this discussion. These practitioners are popularly categorised as Herbalists, Psychic Healers, and Medical Herbalists (those trained at KNUST and awarded degrees in Herbal Medicine), since traditional medicine is not a unified practice (Anyinam, 1997). What these practitioners all have in common is the use of herbs, whether standardised or not, for the treatment of diseases despite other unique practices, as in the case of Psychic Healers who add Spiritism to their practice.

According to the TMPC, as of 2017, a total number of 9287 indigenous practitioners were registered and issued certificates and/or licenses to practice; 6140 were Herbalists, 2996 were Psychic Healers, and 151 were Medical Herbalists. In 2017 alone about 1717 indigenous practitioners were registered by the Council and issued certificates to practice, while 1617 practice premises were registered and licensed. During the same period, 1160 licensed premises had their licenses renewed.

Although the above numbers may appear high, they fall far short of Ghana's needs, considering the existing gaps in healthcare provision in the country. As of 2019, Ghana had a total of 3236 biomedical doctors. This puts the density of medical doctors in Ghana at 1.4 per 10,000 inhabitants as of 2020 (Sasu, 2022), falling short of the WHO-required standard of 1:1000 (Tarlue, 2022). Despite the huge potential of traditional medicine to complement biomedicine in achieving universal health coverage in the country, the government has yet to offer the needed support to unleash this potential. Evidence suggests that there are over 15,000 recognised practitioners and facilities across the country offering Traditional, Alternative and Complementary medical care (Numo, 2019), yet bringing them on board to augment medical care has become difficult.

Additionally, statistics provided by the TMPC reveal an imbalance in the regional distribution of registered practitioners. They are clustered in the populous regions of the southern sector of the country, namely Greater Accra, Ashanti, Brong Ahafo, Central, Western, and Eastern regions, with a few from Northern Ghana (Missodey & Arhinful, 2022). This occurrence could be attributed to the fact that regulatory activities are on the low side in the Northern sector of the country due to resource constraints, as well as to capitalist ideas which focus on cities as the backbone of the global economy (Dronova & Brunn, 2018). In the words of the TMPC's Public Relations Officer, "The last time the Council had financial clearance to employ personnel for its activities was in 2011 and that was for twenty personnel to man regional offices and others in the head office for monitoring. Considering the size of Ghana, and the number of practitioners, this number is woefully inadequate" (Numo, 2019).

Due to these trends, many practitioners move to urban centres to maximise their gains in the industry. As a result, the practice of traditional medicine in Ghana no longer depends solely on expertise. In the urban centres, owners of the means of production enter into partnerships with healers—who remain the main sources of knowledge for the production of standardised herbal medicines, and yet know next to nothing about the production processes. In the end, the healers are alienated from the knowledge they give out. This phenomenon gives rise to another category of practitioners who are mostly labelled as "Manufacturers": they go into business specifically to manufacture, but rely on the knowledge of others for manufacturing. Mr. Soko, a traditional healer based in Accra, lamented thus:

> The pressure to use modern methods is a worry because those who do not have enough knowledge in the field are the ones who have money to acquire licenses, manufacture, and package their products nicely. But those who know and have the skills cannot afford the money to go through the processes and to also package their products according to the professional standards required by regulation.

This modern trend, some have argued, detaches traditional medicine from its cultural heritage, trading it for money: that is, by turning it into a commodity and separating the producer from the prescriber (Banerjee & Mitra, 2012; Danso, 2005; Harilal, 2009; Kloos, 2015). This phenomenon arises because some modern practitioners establish expensive and well-equipped herbal clinics where the manufactured products are prescribed. With evidence from the field, this chapter argues that the commoditisation of traditional medicine also alienates the source of knowledge, which is the traditional healer, from processes of production and prescription. It alienates the traditional healers from their knowledge and empowers the prescriber, thus establishing a kind of professionalism that discards the traditional holistic methods of healthcare in favour of more technocratic and formal approaches to health provision (Morantz-Sanchez, 2005). This affirms the assertion that modern social life is pervaded by standardisation, and often linked with quantification and formal representation (Star & Lampland, 2009).

Inadvertently, the provision of traditional medicine is transferred from healer-specific locations to distribution outlets, and systematically separates healers from the traditional institutions of social and political power within which their autonomy and authority are established. Regulating traditional knowledge forms within the context of modern bureaucracies and biomedical science (Harilal, 2009; Kim, 2007) has led to contestations and struggles over the years in Ghana's medical sphere. Healers contest this new trend, and question why they have to practice their "own traditional knowledge" in the context of a professionalism which is counterproductive as far as traditional healing principles are concerned. Scholars have pointed out that standards are relative and thereby vary in their meaning and impact on groups and individuals across socio-cultural spaces (Star & Lampland, 2009). Therefore, Ghanaian healers hold the view that tradition has standards which cannot be measured accurately using the "scales" of modern science, which was developed in a different social milieu. Papa Kwame, a healer, expressed his view in this manner:

> I don't use other people's products at my clinic. I have only four manufactured products on the market, but if I get a thousand patients, I will have different remedies for each of their ailments. We have our own standards. Our forefathers used the herbs together with different methods yesterday and they were efficacious. Why can't we work with the same standards today? Why are we required to subject our herbs to analysis and turn them into modern drugs and items for sale before they can be used? I don't trust that system. They steal our knowledge.

Nana Ansah, a psychic healer, echoed this view:

> Some herbs may be used for medicines which can never be replicated. If you try it, you will not succeed because I spoke to the plants before harvesting them. You may doubt it but it's a principle and truth in traditional healing. I may have to teach you. But there is what we call "ma hyira so ama wo" (you have my blessing to use the herbs for healing) and "ma kyerɛ wo kɛkɛ" (you have only been told the uses of the herbs).

Hence protesting healers hold on to the cultural values attached to their practices, and the belief that healing is not imbued in the chemical properties of plants but in the hands of healers, as expressed by Nana Ansah. Others have argued that professionalism forges new relations among governments, citizens, and corporate interests. Thus the health of the public is viewed through the lens of the market, and transforms the landscape in which Africans address illness, care for bodies, and seek assistance for their misfortunes (Langwick, 2015).

Besides the struggle in getting healers to accept the established standards, there is evidence that the activities of the TMPC and the FDA regarding regulation overlap. This has become a source of tension between the two regulatory bodies. While the TMPC licenses practitioners, as well as their practices, the FDA is interested in the herbal products and the premises where they are produced and stored. Healers, most of the time, are the manufacturers of their herbal products, and due to resource constraints are unable to separate the clinic from the manufacturing site. In effect, the same premise is registered differently by the two regulators because it is used for activities which are considered separate under the regulations. This is a worry for healers because they think it entails a duplication of mandates.

A critical analysis of the gaps existing in the implementation of these regulatory policies reveals a lack of effective communication between the two implementing agencies, as they both fall under the MOH, which has oversight responsibilities. While they have not been able to deal with these challenges to ease the pressure on healers, the regulators have dissenting views, holding healers responsible. Mr. Adam, an FDA official, explained that, "in most cases, the same healer acts as the researcher, manufacturer, 'herbal doctor' and nurse; and interestingly has the manufacturing facility and clinic at the same premises." So, Mr. Adam emphasised, "Since the herbal doctor is manufacturing within the premises of the clinic, both institutions have the right to pursue their mandate without hindrance." However, further investigations show that the mistrust healers have for regulators and plant medicine researchers makes it difficult to entrust aspects of their practices to other experts in the name of professionalism.

While the above phenomenon is largely experienced in urban areas, the industry remains less developed in rural areas, where the majority of healers are located, and is sometimes described as a dying practice (Anyinam, 1987). Dronova and Brunn (2018) described cities as the initiators of global change and as such as the backbone of the global economy. This phenomenon reshapes cities, making them suitable to fulfil the demands of capitalism. To ascertain the validity of the above assertion, some data were gathered in parts of the Upper West, Savannah, and Northern regions. Apart from one practitioner, all the others contacted were oblivious to the activities of the FDA and the TMPC. They engage their clients through the traditional modes of practice, maintaining the cultural distinctions of their respective traditions. Neindoo, a 42-year-old healer said: "Our ancestors taught us. We didn't go to school but they gave us visions to teach and practice." Essentially, what this means is that in place of regulatory standards, healers draw on different registers to authenticate and legitimise practices. Evidence suggests that the traditional medicine landscape of Ghana has various categories of healers, as there are different therapies and approaches to healing. They are mainly categorised as herbalists, spiritual healers (priests/priestesses of deities, diviners, exorcists), faith healers, bonesetters, and traditional birth attendants, among others. Some are also identified as specialists: for example, bonesetters are a specialist group of healers (Rasmussen, 1998; Senah et al., 2001; Tabi et al., 2006). They acquired their healing knowledge and authority through inheritance, divine calling, apprenticeship, and impartation as a result of good behaviour or kindness. The means of knowledge acquisition becomes the authority on which healers rely to practice, as it is believed that healing knowledge is bequeathed to the living by the ancestors and other spirit beings. Neindoo further explained:

> My forefathers were spiritual healers but when my last grandfather died the practice was neglected because no one was interested. I was a tour guide for many years before I was summoned to come back home and revive the practice which had been neglected for about 14 years. I am 42 years old but I have been in this practice for only 5 years. The number of years in practice does not matter because my call was divine. No one teaches me what to do.

Indeed, no one teaches healers what to do once the call to practice is authentic, and apprentices glory in their authority. This somehow resonates with the assertion that standards do not develop acontextually and are relative to social worlds, thereby resulting in varying impact and meanings. However, females are still constrained in responding to calls to practice medicine by several socio-cultural factors, which has been revealed in the registers generated on traditional medicine practitioners, practices, and products. The chapter now turns attention to the gender dynamics in Ghana's traditional medicine landscape.

5.4 Gender Dynamics

Out of the 6140 registered herbalists mentioned above, an estimated number of 1188 are females, which represents approximately 22.11% of the total number. The remaining 4185 are males, constituting 77.88% of the total number. Only about 270 of the 2996 Psychic Healers are females, whereas males account for about 2720. That represents, approximately, 9.15% and 90.79% of female and male practitioners respectively. For Medical Herbalists, there are 40 females and 111 males, giving approximate percentages of 26.32 and 73.69 respectively. This gender disparity in favour of men does not come as a surprise, as it reflects patterns of poor female representation in various professions across the globe.

In the United States, for example, women were not allowed into the medical profession until the Antebellum Health Reform Movement in the early nineteenth century, which fought to bring women into the public domain, and also championed the idea that health is also a female responsibility (Morantz-Sanchez, 2005). Over the years, selection, especially into science-biased fields of study and careers, has always been skewed towards males in Ghana (UNICEF, 2021). Various socio-cultural and economic reasons have been cited to explain this age-old development. Atuahene and Owusu-Ansah (2013) rightly argue that the systemic factors cited to explain gender-based inequities decades ago in the country remain relevant in recent times. Among these factors are socio-cultural considerations, gendered social practices within households, financial difficulties associated with women's education, a lack of role models for girls in schools, and a hostile school environment (Atuahene & Owusu-Ansah, 2013).

In addition, the colonial legacy of assigning public and private roles to males and females respectively has also contributed to entrenching this phenomenon. Women were, and are still expected, to be content with managing aspects of social life that are considered feminine, like teaching young children, safekeeping social morality, offering moral and religious support to vulnerable groups, housekeeping, and nurturing the family (Morantz-Sanchez, 2005). Females are not trusted with the capacity to combine the hard and soft skills of medical practice—the science and sympathy of the practice respectively, be it traditional or conventional (Atuahene & Owusu-Ansah, 2013; Morantz-Sanchez, 2005; UNICEF, 2021). However, women's right to participate in public life should not be based on any of the above considerations, but should stem from the principles of equity, justice, and job satisfaction that contribute to human development (Morantz-Sanchez, 2005). The global quest for new areas of medicine, as well as the drive to produce standardised, high-quality, safe, and efficacious traditional medicinal products make it imperative for more women to be given the opportunity to bring their expertise on board.

5.5 Standardisation of Products

In Ghana, the institution mandated by law to verify the purity of drugs produced from herbs is the Centre for Plant Medicine Research (ACT 833, 2011). This cause has been championed by the Centre since 1975 based on the pioneering works of its founder, Dr. Oko Ampofo. In the early days of the Centre's operations, the medications came in the form of decoctions which were simply boiled, stored in plastic drums, and dispensed to patients in large containers. The dispensation of decoctions continued until the introduction of official standards meant to guide the preparation and packaging of herbal medications. Dr. Ampofo indicated that he started the process of standardisation by taking the plants to the Department of Botany at the University of Ghana for botanic identification, potency, safety, and efficacy.

As a first step, standard formulae were developed for the preparation of herbal medicines for various indications, and the steps for preparation were outlined to ensure standardisation. The medications thus produced had to undergo laboratory analysis in three critical areas: microbiology, pharmacology, and phytochemistry. The microbiological assay determines how wholesome and efficacious the product is; the pharmacological assay determines the margin of safety of the product, and the wider the margin of safety, the safer the product; and the phytochemical assay indicates whether the product is plant-based or not, as well as the pH level. All these are to fall within the acceptable limits provided by the WHO.

Evidence from the field suggests that before the Centre's establishment, the current form of production, as well as the preclinical safety and toxicity studies of the products mentioned above, were not components of traditional medical practice. These practices became popular with the initial works of Ampofo. Before then, most traditional healers just gave out plant parts to their clients to boil, and the dosage was arbitrarily measured. This accordingly led to standardisation issues (Craig, 2011; Evans-Anfom, 1984). Elaborating on this point, Miss Adwoa, a research scientist at the Centre, opined:

> Using the modern trend has improved the quality of the herbal products we are using now. We know the exact dose that the patient should take that won't have any toxicity or serious consequences. Before, practitioners will tell you to take one cup but people have different sizes of cups. We train herbalists to be able to conform to modern trends so that they don't lose out and don't end up harming people.

As earlier indicated, the registration and certification of all foods and drugs are solely the responsibility of the FDA. Since herbal medicines are also registered as drugs, the preamble to the regulation of drugs stipulated in Act 851 also applies to all herbal medicinal products. No one is allowed to manufacture, sell, prepare, store, or transport herbal medicine unless it is registered by the FDA. In this regard, the FDA has worked in collaboration with the Centre to help practitioners meet the standards of regulation. In pursuance of Section 118 of Act 851, the FDA prepared some guidelines in 2013 with the sole aim of guiding applicants on the procedure of registering traditional medicinal products in Ghana. Applicants are expected to familiarise themselves with this document and the law supporting it before completing the registration form. Applicants are also required to present an analysis report from the Centre or any of the recent testing facilities, a sample of the product, and a registration fee of GHS 360 (about 36 USD).

A list obtained from the Herbal Medicine Unit of the FDA shows that as of 2022, 400 locally manufactured herbal medicines were registered. The details available on each product include product name, dosage form, applicant/manufacturer, indication, and date of product expiry. These products come in various dosage forms, including decoctions, capsules, powders, ointments, and balms. It must be noted that the indications for these products are limited to acute conditions. Per the FDA's regulations, herbal medicines are not allowed for chronic conditions since it is difficult to conduct clinical trials on them in the country as of now. Some of the common indications include malaria, anaemia, immune system booster, skin infections, coughs, constipation, piles, and menstrual, rheumatic, abdominal, and bodily pains, among others.

However, scholars (Craig, 2011; Harilal, 2009; Kloos, 2008) have argued that the effort to standardise has reduced traditional medicine to the status of pharmaceuticals, the defining feature of modernisation in the practice. In the case of the Centre, modernisation is perceived as combining traditional medical knowledge with modern scientific knowledge in the production of traditional herbal medicine. In Ampofo's own words, "The old method translated into the modern method." With these interventions, healthcare delivery, globally, has been reduced to pharmaceuticals, with an emphasis on the availability, affordability, quality, and safety of drugs (Craig, 2011; Kloos, 2017, 2019). It has drawn herbal medicine production into the global capitalist healthcare market (Kloos, 2017), a phenomenon enabled by neoliberal State policies that became popular in the 1980s (O'Sullivan, 2018). Information gathered from field interviews pointed out that the development of herbal medicine into a modern pharmaceutical industry in Ghana became significant in the 1980s.

5.6 Conclusion

Understanding traditional medical practice in Ghana requires an appreciation of the politics involved in professionalising practitioners and standardising products, as this chapter has demonstrated. Specific policies, such as Act 575, Act 831, and establishing Herbal Medicine departments in the country's higher learning institutions, have proven to be significant steps taken by the State in professionalising the practice. Consequently, traditional medicine has undergone a transformation which differs significantly from the past, albeit not across the board. In this light, practitioner associations leverage their numerical strength to negotiate desired changes and due recognition in the medical landscape of the country, which has been a struggle since colonial times, as the trajectories of development described above have revealed. The generation of statistics turns out to play a significant role in the maintenance and continued existence of the associations.

While quantification—the numerical representation of both practitioners and products—is encouraged in the current regulatory regime, it is a bother, from the perspective of healers, as it leads to the de-traditionalisation of traditional medicine—a kind of commodification isolated from traditional principles of healing. Essentially, medicine is not supposed to be sold, nor is the healer supposed to put money first in their practice. Contrary to this traditional demand, health regulatory policies, which are driven by development agendas and promoted by neoliberalism, alienate traditional systems from their historical, social, and cultural values, presenting them as marketable commodities. However, the cultural, including some magico-religious aspects of the practice, is still adhered to by the majority of healers in the country—largely in the northern and rural settings, where the impact of regulation is felt less, as a result of the unequal distribution of regulatory resources, including personnel. This category of healers often draws on registers of authenticity—divine call, impartation, inheritance, apprenticeships—which are considered quite old-fashioned, but acceptable among users within their catchment.

In Ghana, as in many other jurisdictions, endless questions are raised concerning the safety, quality, and efficacy standards of traditional medicine, despite the available evidence of its effective use over the years. The WHO's traditional medicine strategy maintains that biomedical standards should drive traditional medicine's standards, in order to make it practical and scientific. While creating and implementing new standards is not bad in itself, the processes often go unquestioned despite their ethical implications. The focus is mainly on the goal of standardising, even though the process can be cumbrous and authoritarian. A compelling argument has been made that drug regulatory regimes have failed to consider the difference between traditional medical knowledge and biomedicine in setting quality, safety, and efficacy standards. Traditional medicine researchers agree that a better approach is to consider a translation of the existing traditional standards into modern forms that can make them more appealing and attractive, instead of setting entirely new standards based on biomedical scientific practices.

Given these analyses, it is clear that the impact of external and internal regulatory standards in the mass production of traditional medical remedies is far-reaching, as the transformations therein reflect a detachment from the values upon which the practice is anchored. In conclusion, the chapter reiterates the position that there is no way one can understand traditional medical practice in Ghana without recourse to the statistics generated through regulatory standardising procedures, and the effects of these standards on practitioners, practices, and products.

References

ACT575. (2000). Traditional medicine practice act. *Ministry of Health.*

ACT833. (2011). Centre for plant medicine research act, 2011.

ACT851. (2012). Ghana public health act GPC/A753/350/11/2012, Act 851.

Addae, S. (1996). *History of western medicine in Ghana: 1880–1960.* Durham Academic Press.

Adu-Gyamfi, S. (2010). *A historical study of the impact of colonial rule on indigenous medical practices in Ashante: A focus on colonial and indigenous disease combat and prevention strategies in Kumase, 1902–1957* [Ph.D. thesis, Kwame Nkrumah University of Science and Technology].

Adu-Gyamfi, S. (2015). British colonial reform of indigenous medical practices amongst the Asante people of the Gold Coast, 1930–1960. *African Journal of History and Culture, 7*(2), 57–63.

Agyei-Baffour, P., Kudolo, A., Quansah, D. Y., & Boateng, D. (2017). Integrating herbal medicine into mainstream healthcare in Ghana: Clients' acceptability, perceptions and disclosure of use. *BMC Complementary and Alternative Medicine, 17*(1), Article 513.

Ampomah, I. G., Malau-Aduli, B. S., Seidu, A.-A., Malau-Aduli, A. E. O., & Emeto, T. I. (2023). Integrating traditional medicine into the Ghanaian health system: Perceptions and experiences of traditional medicine practitioners in the Ashanti region. *International Health, 15*(4), 414–427.

Anyinam, C. A. (1997). The role of female spiritualists in Africa: Persistance with change. *Canadian Women Studies, 17*(1), 103–106.

Anyinam, C. (1987). Traditional medical practice in contemporary Ghana: A dying or growing "profession"? *Canadian Journal of African Studies/revue Canadienne Des Études Africaines, 21*(3), 315–336.

Anyinam, C. (1989). The social cost of the international monetary fund's adjustment programs for poverty: The case of health care development in Ghana. *International Journal of Health Services, 19*(3), 531–547.

Asante, E., & Avornyo, R. (2013). Enhancing healthcare system in Ghana through integration of traditional medicine. *Journal of Sociological Research, 4*(2), 256–272.

Atuahene, F., & Owusu-Ansah, A. (2013). A descriptive assessment of higher education access, participation, equity, and disparity in Ghana. *SAGE Open, 3*(3), 1–16.

Banerjee, S., & Mitra, A. (2012). Changing landscape of herbal medicine: Technology attributing rennaissance. *International Journal of Pharmacy and Pharmaceutical Sciences, 4*(1), 47–52.

Boateng, M. A., Danso-Appiah, A., Turkson, B. K., & Tersbol, B. P. (2016). Integrating biomedical and herbal medicine in Ghana—Experiences from the Kumasi south hospital: a qualitative study. *Complementary Alternative Medicine, 16*(189), 1–8.

Chary, A., & Sargent, C. (2016). Blending western biomedicine with local healing practices. *AMA Journal of Ethics, 8*(9), 691–697.

Craig, S. R. (2011). Good" manufacturing by whose standards? Remaking concepts of quality, safety, and value in the production of tibetan medicines. *Anthropological Quarterly, 84*(2), 331–378.

Danso, S. A. (2005). The traditional approach to the management of diseases in Ghana. *Legon Journal of Sociology, 2*(2), 69–80.

Droney, D. (2014). Ironies of laboratory work during Ghana's second age of optimism. *Cultural Anthropology, 29*(2), 363–384.

Dronova, O., & Brunn, S. D. (2018). How neoliberal globalization processes are transforming Kyiv's nodal areas. *Urbani Izziv, 29*(2), 96–110.

Evans-Anfom, E. (1984). *Traditional medicine in Ghana: Practice, problems and prospects*. Ghana Academy of Arts and Sciences.

Feng, S., Han, M., Lai, L., Wang, S.-C., & Liu, J.-P. (2017). Research capacity at traditional chinese medicine (TCM) centers in China: A survey of clinical investigators. *Evidence-Based Complementary and Alternative Medicine, 2017*, 1–8.

Harilal, M. S. (2009). 'Commercialising traditional medicine': Ayurvedic manufacturing in Kerala. *Economic and Political Weekly, 44*(16), 44–51.

Isola, O. I. (2013). The "relevance" of the African traditional medicine (alternative medicine) to health care delivery system in Nigeria. *The Journal of Developing Areas, 47*(1), 319–338.

Kim, J. (2007). Alternative medicine's encounter with laboratory science. *Social Studies of Science, 37*(6), 855–880.

Kloos, S. (2008). The history and development of Tibetan medicine in exile. *The Tibet Journal, 33*(3), 15–49.

Kloos, S. (2015). (Im-)potent knowledges. preserving 'traditional' Tibetan medicine through modern science. In A. B. G. Mackenthun (Ed.), *Fugitive knowledges: The preservation and loss of knowledge in cultural contact zones* (pp. 123–142). Waxmann Verlag.

Kloos, S. (2017). The pharmaceutical assemblage: Rethinking Sowa Rigpa and the herbal pharmaceutical industry in Asia. *Current Anthropology, 58*(6), 693–717.

Kloos, S. (2019). Humanitarianism from below: Sowa Rigpa, the traditional pharmaceutical industry, and global health. *Medical Anthropology, 39*(2), 1–15.

Langwick, S. A. (2015). Partial publics: The political promise of traditional medicine in Africa. *Current Anthropology, 56*(4), 493–514.

Le Grand, A., & Wondergem, P. (1990). *Herbal medicine and health promotion: A comparative study of herbal drugs in primary health care*. Royal Tropical Institute.

Marsland, R. (2007). The modern traditional healer: Locating 'hybridity' in modern traditional medicine, southern Tanzania. *Journal of Southern African Studies, 33*(4), 751–765.

Missodey, M., & Arhinful, D. K. (2022). Standardized herbal medicines in Ghana: the construction of a substantial share of the medicine market, especially for malaria. In C. Baxerres & M. Cassier (Eds.), *Understanding drugs markets: An analysis of medicines, regulations and pharmaceutical systems in the global south* (pp. 175–198). Routledge.

Morantz-Sanchez, R. (2005). *Sympathy and science: Women physicians in American medicine*: University of North Carolina Press.

Mpinga, E. K., Kandolo, T., Verloo, H., Bukonda, N. K. Z., Kandala, N.-B., & Chastonay, P. (2013). Traditional/alternative medicines and the right to health: Key elements for a convention on global health. *Health and Human Rights, 15*(1), 44–57.

Numo, B. (2019). Universal health coverage: The role of traditional and complementary medicine. *TMPC News, 1*(1), 10–12.

Nyika, A. (2007). Ethical and regulatory issues surrounding African traditional medicine in the context of HIV/AIDS. *Developing World Bioethics, 7*(1), 25–34.

Nyika, A. (2009). The ethics of improving African traditional medical practice: Scientific or African traditional research methods? *Acta Tropica, 112*, S32–S36.

O'Sullivan, D. (2018). Māori, the state and self-determination in the neoliberal age. In D. Howard-Wagner, M. Bargh, & I. Altamirano-Jiménez (Eds.), *The neoliberal state, recognition and indigenous rights* (Vol. 40, pp. 241–256). ANU Press.

Osseo-Asare, A. B. (2016). Writing medical authority: The rise of literate healers in Ghana, 1930–1970. *Journal of African History, 57*(1), 69–91.

Rasmussen, S. J. (1998). AMAGAL: Medicine, healing and power in t'uareg care-giving discourse. *Nomadic Peoples, 2*(1\2), 150–174.

Sasu, D. D. (2022). Number of medical doctors in Ghana. *Statista*. Retrieved December 3, 2022, from https://www.statista.com/statistics/1281626/number-of-medical-doctors-in-ghana/

Senah, K. A., Adusei, J. K., & Akor, S. A. (2001). *A baseline study into traditional medicine in Ghana*. Ministry of Health/DANIDA.

Star, S. L., & Lampland, M. (2009). Recokoning with standards. In M. Lampland & S. L. Star (Eds.), *Standards and their stories: How quantifying, classifying, and formalizing practices shape everyday life* (pp. 25–34). Cornell University Press.

Sujatha, V., & Abraham, L. (2009). Medicine, state and society. *Economic and Political Weekly, 44*(16), 35–43.

Tabi, M. M., Powell, M., & Hodnicki, D. (2006). Use of traditional healers and modern medicine in Ghana. *International Nursing Review, 53*, 52–58.

Tarlue, M. (2022). Ghana records improvement in doctor- to-population ratio. *DailyGuide Network*.

Twumasi, P. A. (2005). *Medical systems in Ghana: A study in medical sociology*. Ghana Publishing Corporation.

UNICEF. (2021). *Sparking adolescent girls' participation and interest in Stem*.

Archival Sources

PRAAD, Koforidua, ADM/KD/33/6/77 Ghana Psychic and Traditional Healing Association, 1965.

PRAAD, Koforidua, ADM/KD/31/6/684, Ghana Psychic and Traditional Healing Association, 1963–1964.

PRAAD, Koforidua, ADM/KD 29/6/69, Fetishes and Charms, 1930 PRAAD, Koforidua, ADM/KD 29/6/106, Fetishes, 1937–1945.

PRAAD, Koforidua, ADM/KD, 33/6/291, Akwapim South District 7 Year Development Plan 1964.

PRAAD, Koforidua, ADM/KD/33/6/113, Dangerous Trees, 1948–1951.

PRAAD, Koforidua, ERG 1/8/4 Tetteh Quashie Memorial Hospital, Mampong, Eastern Region.

PRAAD, Koforidua, ERG 1/1/44, Development Projects in the Eastern Region, 1972–1977.

PRAAD, Koforidua, ERG 1/8/6, Medical Services in Rural Areas, 1953–1974.

PRAAD, Koforidua, ERG 5/1/31, Koforidua Hospital, 1963.

PRAAD, Accra, ADM 4/3/115, Report of Commission of Enquiry into the Kwame Nkrumah Properties, 1966.

J.H. Kwabena Nketia Archive, University of Ghana, Legon, Accra, IAS/3/1/44, Nkrumah Papers, No date.

PART III

Health Records and the Politics of Standardisation

CHAPTER 6

Hepatitis B Virus Infection and the Ghanaian Healthcare Worker: Risk, Standardisation, and Disease Prevention

Vivian Efua Senoo-Dogbey, Florence Naab, and Lillian Akorfa Ohene

6.1 Introduction

Hepatitis B Virus (HBV) infection is a life-threatening disease. Globally, the infection has been identified as the most common chronic infection afflicting humans (Trepo et al., 2014). HBV is a blood-borne infection that is efficiently transmitted through exposure to contaminated blood and body fluids. HBV is one of the blood-borne pathogens most frequently transmitted to Healthcare Workers (HCWs). This characteristic

The authors have no conflicts of interest to declare that are relevant to the content of this article.

V. E. Senoo-Dogbey (✉) · F. Naab · L. A. Ohene
School of Nursing and Midwifery, University of Ghana, Accra, Ghana
e-mail: vesenoo-dogbey@ug.edu.gh

A. Thiel and S. A. Ntewusu (eds.), *The Social Life of Health Data*,
https://doi.org/10.1007/978-981-97-3500-6_6

of the virus is the basis for its recognition as a significant occupational hazard for HCWs worldwide (Coppola et al., 2016).

The consequences of HBV infection are dire, including liver cirrhosis and hepatocellular carcinoma, also called liver cancer. Unfortunately, preventing HBV infection among HCWs has been suboptimal, especially in Sub-Saharan Africa, where the disease is highly endemic. In these areas, there is a high infection transmission rate, and a high disease burden among the general population that HCWs serve. Occupational transmission of the disease to HCWs is equally high, requiring HBV prevention to be prioritised. For these reasons, systems and programs must be instituted to support HCWs in adhering to the recommended strategies for preventing exposure and subsequent infections. A robust and sensitive HBV disease surveillance system in health facilities is needed for effective risk assessment, and for evaluation of the effectiveness of HBV prevention intervention efforts in health facilities. This book chapter argues that standardisation of data collection systems and procedures is a core component of such efforts, yet requires significant work to be achieved. The chapter scrutinises the practices regarding HBV disease surveillance, standardisation of data collection procedures, and use of data for decision-making regarding HBV prevention activities at the health facility level and higher in the Ghanaian healthcare system. To do so, it discusses the risk level of Ghanaian HCWs for HBV infection, and discusses the evidence available on the translation of risk to actual infections. It compares individual HCW and facility-level practices regarding pre-exposure and post-exposure prophylaxis for HBV with recommended practices outlined by the WHO, the Center for Disease Control and Prevention (CDC), and other international health organisations. It lastly describes the evidence-based preventive practices recommended, as well as the level of adherence to these recommendations for HBV prevention among HCWs.

6.2 Hepatitis B Virus Infection and the Ghanaian Healthcare Worker: The Degree of Risk and the Evidence of Actual Infections

Hepatitis B virus (HBV) infection has long been recognised as an occupational hazard to HCWs worldwide. With significant concerns for developing countries such as Ghana, where the protection of HCWs does not appear on the list of healthcare priorities (Sagoe & Pearson, 2001), the challenges associated with HCW protection can be enormous. In these areas, there remains a significant risk of transmission of HBV to HCWs. The main factors influencing the risk of HCWs over a lifetime career, according to Beltrami et al. (2000), include the following:

- the number and types of blood contacts experienced by the HCW;
- the prevalence of blood-borne pathogen infection among patients treated by the HCW; and
- the risk of transmission of infection after a single blood and body fluid contact.

Extrapolating these factors carefully to the Ghanaian context, it is evident that HCWs in Ghana stand a greater risk of acquiring HBV because of their constant interaction with patients, which is imposed by the numerous healthcare services and procedures they perform. For example, occupational blood exposure, mainly through percutaneous injuries, is unacceptably high among Ghanaian HCWs, with prevalence rates of 47% and 29.7% reported in the last five years (Appiagyei et al., 2021; Obirikorang et al., 2018). HBV is highly endemic in Ghana, with the prevalence of the disease among the general population exceeding 8%, as reported by Ofori-Asenso and Agyeman (2016). HBV has also been identified as the blood-borne pathogen with the highest rate of transmissibility, even compared to Human Immunodeficiency Virus (HIV) and Hepatitis C virus (Hepatitis B Foundation, 2023).

The risk of HBV among Ghanaian HCWs has also shown a correlation with some sociocultural and occupational factors. In many healthcare settings in Ghana, there is a high demand for injections, and a subsequent high injection use rate derived from the belief that injectables are more effective than other treatments (Bosu & Ofori-Adjei, 2000). This practice compels HCWs to prescribe injectables and use these preparations to treat various diseases, thereby increasing their risk of percutaneous injuries and exposures.

The Ghanaian HCW's risk for HBV is also increased by the periodic shortages of Personal Protective Equipment (PPE), which have been identified as a great barrier to the practice of Standard Prevention (SPs), which is an important strategy used to decrease contact with blood and body fluids and therefore the risk of exposure to HBV and subsequent infection by the virus (Akagbo et al., 2017).

The high susceptibility among HCWs to HBV infection in Low-Middle-Income Countries (LMICs) and, for that matter, Ghana, has also been linked to inadequate HBV vaccination coverage, and a lack of knowledge about post-exposure prophylaxis (PEP) measures (Afihene et al., 2015; Senoo-Dogbey, 2021, 2022). Unacceptable practices such as careless handling of contaminated objects, reuse of inadequately sterilised medical equipment, and improper or unsafe waste disposal systems, further aggravate the problem and increase the risk and susceptibility of HCWs to HBV (Taneja & Biswal, 2006).

Unlike in the past, research efforts have now revealed an accurate picture regarding the burden of HBV infection among Ghanaian HCWs, an indication of risk being translated into actual infections. Within various categories and professional groups of HCWs, seroprevalence studies have reported 1%, 5.9%, and 6.7% from facilities located in the Central, Greater Accra, and Volta Regions of the country, respectively (Obiri-Yeboah et al., 2019; Senoo-Dogbey et al., 2023; Tawiah et al., 2022). Ironically, these high seroprevalence reports are from regions identified by a nationwide cross-sectional review of in-hospital HBV testing data as having the lowest seroprevalence and burden of HBV in Ghana (Nartey et al., 2022). The issues of poor exposure reporting practices, lack of standardisation in data collection and management, and lack of seroprevalence studies, hinder an accurate quantification of the burden of HBV among HCWs in some regions of Ghana, especially the northern regions. In the absence of HCW-specific prevalence data, we rely on a nationwide prevalence study that reported an HBV prevalence of 15.6–22.7% among the general population in the northern sector of the country. It is now obvious that the burden of HBV among HCWs in these northern regions of Ghana would be equally high, given that the risk of infection in HCWs parallels the high prevalence of HBV infection in the patient population being served (Pappas & Fisher, 1985).

Having a standardised system of HBV exposure notification or reporting, and accurate data collection and analysis of exposure data, helps to avoid the use of proxy indicators that may be inaccurate or incomplete as a basis for decision-making about HCW safety and protection from HBV.

6.3 Hepatitis B Preventive Practices among Healthcare Workers in Ghana: Evidence of Inadequacies and Suboptimal Practices

Hepatitis B virus infection prevention interventions are implemented at two levels: the individual healthcare worker level, and the facility or institutional level.

6.3.1 *Individual-Level Practices*

Vaccination against HBV is a cost-effective strategy for achieving HBV control, and it has been strongly recommended by the WHO to be used by HCWs and persons at risk of exposure to HBV. Even though Ghanaian HCWs have a high-risk perception of HBV infection (Senoo-Dogbey & Wauku, 2022), practices regarding the prevention of HBV among this population are suboptimal. For example, HBV vaccination coverage among HCWs of 53.4%, 44.2%, and 44.8%, respectively, has been reported from the southern, middle, and northern sectors of the country (Ansa et al., 2019; Konlan et al., 2016; Osei et al., 2019). This is evidence that a high proportion of HCWs are not seroprotected amidst the high levels of risk of exposure and infection.

In resource-poor settings where the HBV disease burden is high and HBV vaccination coverage among HCWs is suboptimal, good knowledge of post-exposure prophylaxis (PEP) for HBV is essential for adequate adherence to PEP management programs. In Ghana, there is also evidence to show that not all HCWs have adequate knowledge of PEP for HBV, such that some HCWs did not know of the existence of PEP, while others believed that antiretroviral drugs used as PEP for HIV are equally effective against HBV (Konlan et al., 2016, Senoo-Dogbey, 2022, Tiko, 2023). Studies in Ghana reported that only 65.4% of HCWs knew of the designated exposure reporting pathways, and that only 17.9% of exposed HCWs utilised PEP protocols (Babanawo et al., 2019; Suglo et al., 2021). Compliance with Standard Precautions (SPs) is the hallmark of healthcare practice, and prevents direct contact with blood and body fluids. Studies performed in Ghana showed that many HCWs were noncompliant with SP practices; for example, a study found that only half of the study respondents protected themselves against blood and body fluids during patient care procedures, and only 30.7% complied with infection prevention guidelines (Akagbo et al., 2017; Kondor, 2021).

These suboptimal practices reported from many studies indicate inadequacies in individual-level preventive practices against HBV among Ghanaian HCWs.

Even though routine data collection on occupational health and safety in health facilities via the District Health Information Management System requires the reporting of HBV vaccination and post-exposure prophylaxis use, there is significant underreporting, incomplete data, poor data quality, and non-use of data for decision-making at the various levels of the healthcare system. Perhaps proper standardisation of data on individual-level HBV preventive practices could have identified the deficiencies and gaps, and initiated discussions by policymakers and stakeholders to address the problem.

6.3.2 *Institutional/Facility Level Practices*

Following the recognition of HBV as a blood-borne infection that can be transmitted via occupational exposures, health institutions worldwide have been mandated to organise and implement infection-prevention strategies to ensure that all HCWs are adequately protected (Zingg et al., 2015). Yet reports indicate that governance and leadership in health facilities regarding HBV infection prevention in resource-poor settings such as Ghana are unavailable or non-functional. For example, not all health facilities have occupational health and safety and infection prevention committees to drive HBV-prevention efforts in Ghana. This has mainly contributed to deficiencies in HBV prevention in Ghanaian health facilities. These deficiencies, according to Senoo-Dogbey et al. (2023), are:

- Facilities do not have supplies and logistics such as the HBV vaccine and HBIG or HBV testing kits. Hence, HBV vaccination, assessment of exposed HCWs and source patients, and PEP management programs, are unavailable or non-functional;
- Systems and pathways for exposure reporting are unclear or unavailable for exposure reporting;
- Guidelines and protocols for HBV PEP management are unavailable in facilities; and
- HBV prevention is not integrated into routine in-service training and HCW education programs.

These issues present serious gaps, because good leadership and governance in the health system involves ensuring the existence of policy frameworks combined with effective oversight, coalition building, regulation, attention to system design, and accountability (Manyazewal, 2017). Therefore, these health facility system failures or inadequacies can potentially compromise the health, safety, and protection of HCWs, especially in settings where the risk of exposure to HBV is very high.

A well-functioning health system with a good health information system ensures the production, analysis, dissemination, and use of reliable and timely information on health determinants, health system performance, and health status (Manyazewal, 2017). In the absence of these factors, the goal of HBV prevention among HCWs will not be fully realised.

The fundamental causes of these facility-level gaps in HBV-prevention can be linked to poor data standardisation resulting from deficiencies in data collection and use in the Ghanaian health system. WHO health information systems have four key functions: data generation; data compilation; analysis and synthesis; and communication and use for action (Borghi & Brown, 2022). In the absence of good data standardisation in the health system, policymakers and stakeholders may not appreciate the magnitude of the deficiencies in HBV prevention programs.

6.4 Standardisation, Documentation, and Use of Data for Monitoring Exposures and HBV Prevention Activities Among Healthcare Workers in Ghana

Even though the occupational health and safety policy of the Ghana Health Services mandates active surveillance of all health and safety issues of HCWs, exposure to blood-borne pathogens and uptake of preventive practices are not standardised or streamlined across health facilities; instead, a passive surveillance approach to exposure notification and documentation is adopted and practised in most health settings, which is characterised by a high level of liberality and flexibility in the notification or reporting and documentation of HCW exposures (World Health Organization, 2014).

Reliable information from data is key to decision-making across health system building blocks. Data on occupational exposures is essential for planning preventive measures. It also helps to identify important areas needing attention. To be able to design more targeted prevention mechanisms and related policies, it is recommended to carefully analyse and interpret data. Standardisation allows for data from varied sources to be processed, analysed, and compared more efficiently and accurately. This provides a common set of measures of occupational health and safety that can be compared and monitored over time, and utilised for establishing State priorities and prevention initiatives.

Occupational health and safety data standardisation and management are essential in health facilities to identify and assess risk, track and evaluate the effectiveness of facility-level safety and infection prevention programs, and finally, provide a basis for decisions about how to improve HCW safety within a facility, district, or even the entire nation. Health facilities need an organised system to systematically collect data on occupational exposures. Health facilities maintain incident logbooks in which needle sticks, sharps injuries, and other forms of exposure are recorded by Infection Prevention and Control (IPC) focal persons (Lori et al., 2015). A post-exposure prophylaxis record, which is also filled out by a member of the IPC committee, also serves as documentation of any post-exposure laboratory assessment and treatment regime started for the exposed employee.

For example, a study in Ghana that assessed the occurrence of exposures and use of post-exposure prophylaxis among nurses, found that the data collection system for occupational exposures was notably skewed towards highly-resourced and donor-supported HIV surveillance systems. The study reported that little or no attention was given to HBV, even though HBV is much more transmissible than HIV in the healthcare setting (Lori et al., 2015).

The District Health Information Management System (DHIMS II) is a comprehensive system for capturing, reporting, and analysing health data for the healthcare ecosystem in Ghana and in many other countries around the world. The DHIMS II is a typical example of standardising data collection, analysis, and utilisation across many health systems. This is because this information system makes use of Standard Operation Procedures (SOPs), standard forms for data capture, standardised reporting and data collection procedures, and standardised processes for data analysis. In Ghana, this system has been operational since 2012, and is available in all 216 health districts (Gyaase & Bright, 2019). It has been credited with the capability to collect, process, report, and use health information and knowledge to influence policy and decision-making. Unlike in the past, when paper-based reporting was practised, health facilities currently have the mandate to provide monthly reports on occupational health and safety issues of HCWs by directly and electronically entering data into the DHIMS II database. Despite the positive features described above, the DHIMS II in Ghana is characterised by issues with poor data quality, poor timeliness, and low information usage with poor feedback, all of which have been identified as major challenges (Adaletey et al., 2013). Specifically, for occupational health and safety issues, the IPC or occupational health and safety focal persons are responsible for completing the standardised electronic reporting form every month. Unfortunately, the form only has two components or indicators that are specific to HBV infection among HCWs. These indicators cover individual-level HBV prevention practices, namely:

- The number of recipients for HBV post-exposure prophylaxis; and
- The number of recipients for HBV pre-exposure prophylaxis.

Even though the electronic form also has indicators for staff screening, risk assessment, and incidents in healthcare settings, all these other forms are nonspecific and cover HIV, hepatitis C, and even non-communicable diseases. This makes it extremely difficult to measure HBV-specific indicators among HCWs. Perhaps this is one of the reasons why HBV is obscured and relegated to second-class status, such that stakeholders and policymakers are not fully informed about the burden it imposes and the possible consequences among the Ghanaian HCW population.

For example, a careful examination of HBV-specific country-level data reported in the DHIMS II database between 2019 and 2022 revealed massive underreporting of pre- and post-exposure prophylaxis use for HBV—which are both important indicators of the level of exposure and risk mitigation—as well as of vaccination coverage, which is an important HBV preventive measure among HCWs.

Table 6.1 shows data obtained from the DHIMS II database for the whole country for the year 2019–2022. The data presented for 2019 alone shows that only two HCWs in the whole country reported exposures and received HBV PEP. This is contrary to research findings from a study that recruited HCWs from five facilities in only one region in Ghana in that same year (2019), and reported that seven participants who

Table 6.1 HBV pre- and post-exposure prophylaxis use among Ghanaian HCWs reported in the DHIMS II database (*Source* DHIMS-Ghana Health Service)

HBV indicators	2019	2020	2021	2022
Number of recipients - Hepatitis B (Postexposure prophylaxis)	2	3	37	19
Number of recipients - Hepatitis B (Preexposure prophylaxis)	1	7	71	84

were exposed to HBV received PEP (Senoo-Dogbey, 2021, 2022). This disparity in data presented in the national database provides grounds to suggest that there is an underreporting of HBV indicators for HCWs in Ghana.

Anecdotal evidence from District Health Directorates in Ghana also revealed that the annual and half-year performance reviews that provide platforms for discussions on health indicators do not feature occupational health and safety issues in general. More specifically, HBV-related data is also not presented, reviewed or discussed, and hence not utilised for decision-making at the facility, district, and other higher levels in the Ghanaian health system. These observations reflect the widespread challenges of poor standardisation, underreporting, and poor use of data for action in the Ghanaian health system. This observation is in support of the views of Sagoe and Pearson (2001) that the prevention of bloodborne infections, of which HBV is the most efficiently transmitted, does not appear on the agenda of policymakers in developing countries.

This failure is worrying because accurate data from all health facilities in Ghana could communicate the level of risk of HBV among HCWs to policymakers, stakeholders, and even international partners, and could be the beginning of conversations and dialogue that would provide the funding and support required to protect HCWs.

6.5 Levels of Implementation of Hepatitis B Virus Infection Prevention Practices Among HCWs

Pappas and Fisher (1985) recognised the critical roles of the HCW, as well as the institution or health facility, in implementing HBV preventive strategies. Based on the identification of these roles, the authors outlined two major approaches for the prevention of HBV transmission among HCWs. These approaches include (1) the institutional or facility-level approach, and (2) the individual HCW-level approach.

6.5.1 Institutional/Facility-Level HBV Prevention Approach

The institutional-level approach to HBV prevention begins with hospital or facility-level governance and leadership for HBV prevention. It involves the establishment of the Infection Prevention and Control (IPC) and the Occupational Health and Safety (OHS) Committees. The facility-level approach also entails the establishment of programs and systems, the provision of guidelines, protocols, logistics, and supplies and the establishment of disease surveillance systems. Evidence from other studies has shown that the establishment of institutional-level approaches has contributed significantly to HCW and patient safety in many healthcare settings (Garay et al., 2023; Świtalski et al., 2022; Yassi et al., 2013). In contrast, in Ghana, an audit of 255 health facilities to assess the establishment of these committees and systems to drive HBV prevention programs reported widespread inadequacies in their constitution, along with unavailable or non-functional committees in many of the health facilities audited (Senoo-Dogbey et al., 2023).

The Infection Control Committee and its Role in HBV Prevention in the Health Facility. The WHO recommends a functional IPC program with a dedicated and trained team in each acute healthcare facility to prevent hospital-acquired infections, through good IPC practices. To successfully run the IPC program, a focal person is needed for a primary care level, and one focal person per 250 beds is recommended at secondary levels. For tertiary-level facilities, a well-functioning team or committee with one focal person per 250 beds is needed (World Health Organization, 2019). The committee is an independent authority within the hospital that solely adopts control measures to prevent the transmission of healthcare-associated infection within the hospital (Far et al., 2001). The committee comprises physicians, nurses, laboratory personnel, infection control practitioners, quality assurance officers, disease control personnel, and epidemiologists. It has been documented that health facilities and hospitals having well-organised IPC committees show significant improvement in both patient and HCW safety, improvement in overall quality of services, lower healthcare costs, and most importantly, reduced mortality and morbidity associated with hospital-acquired infections in both patients and HCWs (Far et al., 2001). Unfortunately, the establishment of IPC committees and the appointment of focal persons is not optimal in the Ghanaian health system. For example, Oppong et al. (2020), in their study of 56 acute healthcare facilities in Ghana, revealed that approximately 28 (50%) facilities had IPC committees comprising IPC personnel, and supporting IPC programs in their facilities; 20 facilities had only IPC focal persons; and eight facilities had no IPC personnel in their facilities.

Perhaps the absence of functional IPC committees and their respective focal persons in the health facilities is what has resulted in poor oversight in the health facilities, leading to the poor reporting of exposures and uptake of preventive measures. Most importantly, the inadequate standardisation of data collection procedures analysis, and utilisation of HBV-related data, which is widespread in Ghana, could result from a lack of good governance and leadership for HBV prevention programs, itself resulting from the absence of these committees and focal persons.

The Occupational Health and Safety Committee and its Role in HBV Prevention in the Health Facility. The Occupational Health and Safety (OHS) committee works with employers and all health professionals to create a healthy and safe work environment by detecting occupational health and safety hazards and developing practical approaches to eliminate or control them.

Ghana does not have a national policy on occupational health and safety management, as the ILO Convention No. 155 (1981) requires (Asumeng et al., 2015). However, the Ministry of Health and the Ghana Health Service, in collaboration with the WHO country office, commissioned the development of a policy and guideline on occupational health and safety for the health sector in 2010 (Ghana Health Service, 2010). Despite the widespread dissemination of this policy, there are still major gaps in its implementation in Ghanaian healthcare facilities (Alhassan & Poku, 2018).

Per Ghana's occupational health and safety policy, the OHS committee is essential for bringing health and safety concerns into the open, focusing attention on them, and recommending ways to correct and resolve them (Ghana Health Service, 2010). It is worth noting that the activities of the committee and its respective focal persons are also aimed at generating quality data on occupational health and safety issues and practices in healthcare facilities. Despite the availability of this policy, not all health facilities in Ghana have OHS committees established (Senoo-Dogbey et al., 2023). The absence of functional committees in health facilities has consequences for the accurate documentation of occupational health and safety activities. This makes it difficult to monitor trends of HBV exposures, for example. Again, decisions on the occupational health and safety of HCWs will not be based on any scientific evidence.

Hepatitis B Virus Disease Surveillance, Data Management, and Data Utilisation for Action. Blood-borne pathogen surveillance systems in health facilities are designed to collect, analyse, interpret, and disseminate information on exposure and infection with HBV and other occupational hazards. The surveillance system is intended to provide information regarding the magnitude and trends of sharps injuries and all forms of exposures to identify devices, procedures, and departments most frequently associated with exposures that should be considered priorities for intervention. The WHO recommends that facilities (especially tertiary-level facilities) have active surveillance systems with enabling structures and supporting resources (dependable laboratories, medical records, trained staff), with timely and regular feedback provided to key stakeholders to lead to appropriate action (World Health Organization, 2019). The surveillance system is designed to promptly identify HCWs who suffer exposure and enrol them in PEP management programs. The surveillance system should also cover a facility-level registry of exposures, PEP prescriptions, and seroconversions, if any, to allow researchers and healthcare professionals to obtain an accurate picture of the current situation, and to evaluate the effectiveness of facility-level policies and interventions.

Data for the surveillance system needs to be very accurate, complete, and timely. Documentation of exposures in the healthcare setting is fundamental for the effective evaluation of HCWs for PEP following an exposure; hence, accuracy, completeness, and timeliness are essential. In collaboration with the IPC committee, the OHS committee is responsible for establishing systems for documenting exposures of all forms among HCWs. The documentation should cover the circumstances leading to the exposure as regards the time, date, type of duty being performed, and the instrument or device involved. The documentation vividly describes the exposure in terms of severity, amount and type of body fluid involved, and type of device causing the exposure, as well as the sociodemographic characteristics of the exposed HCW (Beltrami et al., 2000).

Standardised and universally-accepted case definitions for exposures and infections should be available, coupled with standard forms or tools for data collection. Data analysis needs to be organised locally and as part of a national surveillance system, to determine exposure and HBV disease incidence and prevalence, as well as the epidemiologic characteristics of exposed HCWs (Department of Health of the Republic of Philippines, 2021). Despite the recommendation in Ghana's occupational health and safety policy for health facilities to maintain active surveillance systems for occupational exposures, not all facilities adhere to this recommendation. Active surveillance for occupational exposures is much more skewed to HIV, while HBV and other biological exposures are given little or no attention (Lori et al., 2015).

6.5.2 *Facility-Level Programs for HBV Prevention*

HBV Vaccination Program. According to the Pan American Health Organization Regional Office (2015), employee HBV screening and onsite vaccination programs are critical facility-level approaches to HBV prevention. These programs are championed by the facility's occupational health and safety unit with written policies and protocols to guide their actions. Programs can be integrated into the facility's existing health and safety plans. Health facilities are responsible for adequately allocating human and financial resources to ensure the effective implementation of the programs.

To achieve a successful HBV vaccination program, health facilities are required to provide free onsite vaccination with periodic and repeated reminders to HCWs to ensure completion of all three doses of HB vaccine, and also to monitor immunisation coverage. Again, health facilities are also mandated to provide information and training on occupational risks associated with HBV, and other preventive measures including PEP management of exposed HCWs. Another responsibility of health facilities is to make laboratory services for screening and post-vaccination serological testing available to HCWs (Pan American Health Organization Regional Office, 2015).

In Ghana, available reports indicate that some of these facility-level vaccination programs are unavailable or inadequate. For example, onsite vaccination programs are not available in all cases, such that HCWs make personal arrangements for their pre-employment HBV vaccination, a process characterised by the acquisition of vaccines using byzantine supply chain systems. Also, there is widespread unavailability of post-vaccination surveillance programs to evaluate the effectiveness of HBV vaccination programs (Obiri-Yeboah et al., 2019). There is sufficient evidence that these facility-level factors negatively impact the uptake of HBV prevention practices among HCWs in most resource-poor countries (Ndunguru et al., 2023).

Post-exposure Prophylaxis Management Programs. Vaccination against HBV is the mainstay of HBV prevention among HCWs. However, in settings where HBV vaccination coverage is very low, and exposure to blood and body fluids through percutaneous and mucocutaneous exposures is very high, post-exposure prophylaxis (PEP) becomes essential in protecting HCWs from HBV infection (Senoo-Dogbey, 2021, 2022). The occupational health and safety units of health facilities supported by facility management have the responsibility of ensuring that structures are in place to successfully implement PEP management programs for all exposed HCWs. Guidelines and protocols must be available to guide actions. Clear reporting pathways are needed to allow for timely reporting of exposures (Boden et al., 2016). The occupational health and safety physician, nurse, or a focal person, needs to have the requisite knowledge and skills to perform risk assessment, counsel affected HCWs, prescribe PEP regimens, and provide support and follow-up to exposed HCWs per standard policies and guidelines (Singhal et al., 2009). Laboratory supplies and testing materials should be readily available for timely assessment of affected HCWs and source patients, to permit timely decision-making and timely administration of PEP. Accurate documentation of exposures to existing surveillance systems is essential to provide information for action and evaluate the effectiveness of the PEP program (Pan American Health Organization Regional Office, 2015).

This approach to HBV prevention needs to be standardised in all facilities, especially in endemic regions such as Ghana. The data collection procedures about HBV exposure; uptake of preventive intervention by HCWs; and the ultimate utilisation of this information for health action and decision-making, are key strategies for evaluating the effectiveness of facility-level HBV prevention programs.

Unfortunately, many Ghanaian health facilities lack the necessary structures and systems for exposure reporting and PEP management for exposed HCWs. HCWs in such facilities also have inadequate knowledge of PEP for HBV (Senoo-Dogbey, 2022). For example, in a large regional hospital, structures were available for reporting and PEP management for HIV exposure only (Lori et al., 2015), and HCWs suffering exposure to HBV were wrongly managed or offered antiretroviral agents effective against HIV, rather than immunoglobulin and the HB vaccine recommended for PEP management for HBV (Tiko, 2023). Immunoglobulin for PEP management of exposed HCWs is also unavailable in most facilities (Senoo-Dogbey et al., 2023), making it difficult for HCWs needing immediate PEP management to obtain the expensive immunoglobulin at their own cost. According to Tiko (2023), this is a major barrier to the implementation of PEP management for HBV in Ghanaian Health Facilities.

Infection Prevention and Control Training and Educational Programs. Infection prevention and control (IPC) education and training programs are intended to increase HCWs' knowledge, competency, and practical skills about infectious diseases and their prevention. These programs are generally managed by the IPC program of a facility. Education and training programs should be provided to HCWs initially upon hire or, as part of their orientation, periodically during employment. Annual or periodic refresher training sessions are recommended, especially when policies, protocols, or guidelines have been updated or revised and there is a need for dissemination. IPC training and education are equally needed to address a specific need, such as new job duties or responsibilities, or as a response to a particular infectious disease outbreak (Centers for Disease Control & Prevention, 2013). Infection prevention education and training should have multimodal approaches involving train-the-trainer approaches, e-learning, interactive and practical sessions such as simulation and/or bedside training, as well as feedback mechanisms. Others include in-service mentorship presentations, case studies, and discussions (Department of Health of the Republic of Philippines, 2021).

Specifically, to promote the risk reduction for HBV and occupational transmission of HBV to HCWs, IPC education and training programs in health facilities should mandatorily cover PEP for HBV, exposure reporting pathways, and PEP management of exposed HCWs.

This facility-led education and training for HCWs on infection prevention has been shown to reduce the incidence of exposure to blood-borne pathogens, contribute significantly to the reduction of inappropriate practices by HCWs, and improve adherence to policies regarding infection prevention and control in the health facility (El-leithy, 2013; Opiyo & English, 2010; Zafar et al., 2009).

In Ghana, IPC training has been incorporated into pre-service curricula. In addition, regular in-service training for HCWs in infection prevention and control is widespread (Asiedu et al., 2018; Sunkwa-Mills et al., 2023). However, there is a lack of integration of HBV prevention issues, including PEP management, into many of the IPC training programs (Senoo-Dogbey, 2021, 2022). This is evidenced by the unsatisfactory knowledge of HCWs regarding HBV prevention strategies, especially PEP management of exposed HCWs. The poor integration may have contributed largely to the poor uptake of preventive interventions among Ghanaian HCWs.

The Provision of Written Policies, Guidelines, and Protocols on HBV Infection Prevention and Control. IPC policies are the mainstay in ensuring compliance with best evidence-based practices (Cochrane, 2014). IPC policies should meet international, national, and government standards. This is also true of guidelines, procedures, and protocols that should reflect policy content and the most contemporary evidence for best practices (Chambers et al., 2007). The most up-to-date evidence for best practices should underpin all organisational policies/protocols (Barker, 2013).

Specifically, for HBV prevention, guidelines need to provide clear direction on HBV vaccination, exposure reporting, and PEP management for affected HCWs. These protocols in the immediate work environment of HCWs serve as cues for action for HCWs. Although international guidelines exist to guide HBV prevention actions in health facilities, facilities can adapt these guidelines and develop their indicators to address the specific needs of HCWs. The facility-specific guidelines can streamline the approach to exposure reporting, exposure documentation, and analysis of facility-level data. The adapted guidelines can promote facility- and individual-level HBV prevention interventions in the facility, and provide benchmarks for monitoring and evaluating performance.

Even though these recommendations stated above have been widely disseminated, studies done in the Southern and Northern parts of Ghana reported the absence of protocols and guidelines on HBV prevention in the immediate work environment of HCWs (Senoo-Dogbey et al., 2023a; Tiko, 2023). Some participants in one of these studies reported a complete lack of awareness and knowledge of the protocol for PEP management. This observation is worrying, given that protocols and guidelines facilitate adherence, promote compliance and, most importantly, reduce variations in practice (Irving, 2014).

Provision of Logistics and Supplies for HBV Infection Prevention and Control Activities. To meet basic levels of IPC readiness, healthcare facilities need access to essential supplies and logistics to implement the HBV prevention program effectively. These supplies include soap and water or alcohol-based hand rubs for hand hygiene, proper waste receptacles for safe separation, transportation and disposal of medical waste, and sufficient personal protective equipment (PPE) stocks to protect staff, patients, and visitors.

Specifically, for HBV prevention, health facilities need reasonable and adequate supplies of HBV vaccines and HBIG for effective facility-level vaccination programs and PEP management programs. Additionally, supplies such as laboratory testing kits that are highly sensitive, specific, and rapid are needed for patient and staff evaluation or risk assessment following exposures (Pan American Health Organization Regional Office, 2015).

Regardless of these recommendations, some studies have reported insufficient supplies and non-availability of logistics such as HBV vaccine, immunoglobulin, PPEs, and other supplies for IPC practice in some facilities in Ghana (Akagbo et al., 2017; Senoo-Dogbey et al., 2023a).

Providing adequate, appropriate supplies to health workers in an effective logistics system also increases their professional satisfaction, motivation, and morale. More importantly, a well-supplied facility IPC program can provide high-quality service where HCWs can use their training and expertise fully, directly improving the quality of care for clients, promoting adherence to IPC standards and protocols, and improving overall HCW safety.

6.5.3 *Individual-Level HBV Prevention Approach*

Healthcare workers are significant stakeholders in every facility or hospital's infection prevention program. HCWs are responsible for participating in periodic training programs to receive periodic and regular updates and training on new products, procedures, and protocols regarding their occupational health and safety. Complete adherence to SPs is critical to preventing exposure to potentially infectious biological materials. However, studies have shown that this practice is sub-optimal among Ghanaian HCWs, as among HCWs in other developing countries. For example, a study in Ghana found that only 50% of the participants always adhered to standard precautions protocol (Akagbo et al., 2017).

Specifically, for HBV prevention, there is a need for all HCWs to benefit from facility-level HBV vaccination programs and receive the recommended 3-dose HBV vaccine at the recommended 0,1,6 vaccination schedule. Nevertheless, it has been reported that not all HCWs have benefited from vaccination programs, as HB vaccination coverage is still below 90% (Ansa et al., 2019).

HCWs need to rely on facility-level structures to determine their response to the HBV vaccine by undergoing post-vaccination serological testing two months post-vaccination, and having their antibody levels duly documented per international recommendations (Centers for Disease Control & Prevention, 2013; Pan American Health Organization Regional Office, 2015).

Despite this recommendation, a study done in Ghana found that only 21.3% of HCWs undertook post-vaccination serological testing to assess their immune status post-vaccination (Senoo Dogbey et al., 2023b).

In case of exposure to blood and body fluids with the risk of HBV transmission, HCWs need to immediately report their exposures using the established channels within the facility. The affected HCW ought to avail himself for risk assessment or evaluation for the need for PEP management, and comply with the PEP regimen (HBV vaccine and/or HBIG) and post-PEP care and follow-up that would be prescribed if needed (CDC, 2013; National Center for Immunization Research & Surveillance, 2015). Reports available from southern Ghana indicate that not all HCWs report their exposures. According to Babanawo et al. (2019), only 33.8% of HCWs from a large regional hospital who suffered exposure reported and received the appropriate PEP regimen, an indication of the increasing risk of HBV infection among Ghanaian HCWs.

6.6 Conclusion

Hepatitis B virus is an important occupational hazard for HCWs. The risk of exposure to HBV and its associated disease burden among HCWs in Ghana is still high. In the face of this, the Ghanaian context is facing challenges of insufficient implementation of individual-level preventive strategies including low HB vaccination coverage, inadequate adherence to standard precaution protocols, poor exposure reporting, and suboptimal PEP management practices. There are substantial gaps in health facility-level preventive approaches, which have negatively impacted the individual-level HBV preventive practices recommended for individual HCWs. Some of these facility-level issues include a lack of logistics, protocols, and guidelines, unavailability or non-functionality of IPC and occupational health and safety committees, and insufficient integration of HBV prevention in routine IPC training for HCWs. These gaps have consequences for HCW safety and protection against HBV. All these gaps have been linked to a lack of active surveillance of HBV in health facilities. There are major gaps in the level of data standardisation on exposure patterns, uptake of preventive interventions, and ultimate use of information for decision-making.

While working to reduce the risk and infections among Ghanaian HCWs, HBV disease surveillance and standardisation of data collection procedures are urgently needed to continuously and systematically collect data to monitor progress, and provide a basis for HBV prevention decision-making to promote HCW safety. Data production brings attention to the magnitude of the burden of risk, and of the infections of HBV in HCW populations. Data standardisation provides a basis for prioritising and distributing scarce resources. The use of data allows for a logic of monitoring and evaluation of the effectiveness of preventive interventions. This can be helpful in mobilising HCWs to adopt measures through evidence. However, data itself requires standards and substantial efforts to be collected, analysed, and used in meaningful ways.

References

Adaletey, D. L., Poppe, O., & Braa, J. (2013). Cloud computing for development—Improving the health information system in Ghana. In P. Cunningham & M. Cunningham (Eds.), *IST-Africa 2013 conference proceedings* (pp. 1–9). IIMC International Information Management Corporation.

Afihene, M. Y., Duduyemi, B. M., & Khatib, M. (2015). Knowledge, attitude and practices concerning Hepatitis B infection, among healthcare workers in Bantama, Ghana : A cross-sectional study. *International Journal of Community Medicine and Public Health, 2*(3), 244–253.

Akagbo, S. E., Nortey, P., & Ackumey, M. M. (2017). Knowledge of standard precautions and barriers to compliance among healthcare workers in the Lower Manya Krobo District Ghana. *BMC Research Notes, 10*(1), 1–10.

Alhassan, R. K., & Poku, K. A. (2018). Experiences of frontline nursing staff on workplace safety and occupational health hazards in two psychiatric hospitals in Ghana. *BMC Public Health, 18*(1), 1–12.

Ansa, G. A., Ofori, K., Houphouet, E. E., Amoabeng, A. A., Sifa, J. S., Amenuveve, C. K., & Odame, G. H. (2019). Hepatitis B vaccine uptake among healthcare workers in a referral hospital, Accra. *The Pan African Medical Journal, 33*(96). https://doi.org/10.11604/pamj.2019.33.96.18042

Appiagyei, H., Nakua, E. K., Donkor, P., & Mock, C. (2021). Occupational injuries among health care workers at a public hospital in Ghana. *Pan African Medical Journal, 39*(103). https://doi.org/10.11604/pamj.2021.39.103.23542

Asiedu, A., Ayetey, J., Agblanya, C., Favero, R., Galvin, A., & Asare, K. (2018). *MCSP Ghana : Lessons from a competency-based infection prevention and control (IPC) training approach key findings and recommendations brief*.

Asumeng, et al. (2015). Occupational safety and health issues in Ghana. *International Journal of Business and Management Review, 3*(9), 60–79.

Babanawo, F., Ibrahim, A., Bahar, O. S., Adomah-Afari, A., & Maya, E. (2019). Assessment of knowledge and usage of HIV post exposure prophylaxis among healthcare workers in a regional hospital in Ghana. *Journal of Global Health Reports, 2*, 1–14.

Barker, J. (2013). *Evidence-based practice for nurses and healthcare professionals* (2nd ed., Vol. 1, Issue 1). Sage Publications.

Beltrami, E. M., Williams, I. T., Shapiro, C. N., & Chamberland, M. E. (2000). Risk and management of blood-borne infections in health care workers. *Clinical Microbiology Reviews, 13*(3), 385–407.

Boden, L. I., Petrofsky, Y. V., Hopcia, K., Wagner, G. R., & Hashimoto, D. (2016). Understanding the hospital sharps injury reporting pathway. *American Journal of Industrial Medicine, 118*(24), 6072–6078.

Borghi, J., & Brown, G. W. (2022). Taking systems thinking to the global level: Using the WHO building blocks to describe and appraise the global health system in relation to COVID-19. *Global Policy, 13*(2), 193–207.

Bosu, W. K., & Ofori-Adjei, D. (2000). An audit of prescribing practices in health care facilities of the Wassa West district of Ghana. *West African Journal of Medicine, 19*(4), 298–303.

Centers for Disease Control and Prevention. (2013). *Guide to infection prevention for outpatient settings: Minimum expectations for safe care*. Centers for Disease Control and Prevention.

Chambers, R., Boath, E., & Rogers, D. (2007). *Clinical effectiveness and clinical governance made easy* (4th ed.). Radcliffe Publishing.

Cochrane, J. M. (2014). Are your IPC policies fit for purpose? *Journal of Infection Prevention, 15*(5), 164–168.

Coppola, N., De Pascalis, S., Onorato, L., Calò, F., Sagnelli, C., & Sagnelli, E. (2016). Hepatitis B virus and hepatitis C virus infection in healthcare workers. *World Journal of Hepatology, 8*(5), 273–281.

Department of Health of the Republic of Phillippines. (2021). *National standards in infection prevention and control for health facilities*. Department of Health of the Republic of Phillippines.

El-leithy, B. (2013). Education program about blood born-pathogens transmission on primary health care workers in Ismailia city (an intervention study). *Egyptian Journal of Occupational Medicine, 37*(2), 121–139.

Far, F. E., Marino, C. G., & Medeiros, E. A. (2001). The organization of hospital infection control committees and their importance in Brazil. *The Brazilian Journal of Infectious Diseases, 5*(6), 290–293.

Garay, S., Haeger, M., Kühnlein, L., Sulmann, D., & Suhr, R. (2023). Interventions to enhance safety culture for nursing professionals in long-term care: A systematic review. *International Journal of Nursing Studies Advances, 5*, Article 100119. https://doi.org/10.1016/j.ijnsa.2023.100119

Ghana Health Service. (2010). Occupational health and safety policy and guidelines, ministry of health and ghana health service. Retrieved March 6, 2024, from https://www.moh.gov.gh/wp-content/uploads/2016/02/Occupational-Health-Safety-Policy-Guidelines-for-Health-Sector.pdf

Gyaase, P. O., & Bright, K. (2019). An extension of the information systems success model; A study of district health information management system (DHIMS II) in Ghana. In A. Jamalipour, M. Ruggieri, & J. Zhang (Eds.), *Handbook on ICT in developing countries: Next generation ICT technologies* (pp. 1–318). River Publishers.

Hepatitis B Foundation. (2023). *Hepatitis B facts and figures*. Retrieved March 6, 2024, from https://www.hepb.org/what-is-hepatitis-b/what-is-hepb/facts-and-figures/

Irving, A. V. (2014). *Policies and procedures for healthcare organizations: A risk management perspective—patient safety & quality healthcare*. Patient Safety and Quality Healthcare. Retrieved March 6, 2024, from https://www.psqh.com/analysis/policies-and-procedures-for-healthcare-organizations-a-risk-management-perspective/

Kondor, V. D. (2021). Health worker compliance with infection prevention and control policy in Ghana: A case study of La General Hospital. *Texila International Journal of Public Health, 9*(2), 150–161.

Konlan, K. D., Aarah-Bapuah, M., Kombat, J. M., & Wuffele, G. M. (2016). The level of nurses' knowledge on occupational post-exposure to hepatitis B infection in the Tamale metropolis Ghana. *BMC Health Services Research, 1*(12), 1–15.

Lori, J. R., McCullagh, M. C., Krueger, A., & Oteng, R. (2015). Sharps injuries among emergency department nurses in one tertiary care hospital in Ghana. *International Emergency Nursing, 28*, 14–19.

Manyazewal, T. (2017). Using the World Health Organization health system building blocks through survey of healthcare professionals to determine the performance of public healthcare facilities. *Archives of Public Health, 75*(1), 1–8.

Nartey, Y. A., Okine, R., Seake-Kwawu, A., Ghartey, G., Asamoah, Y. K., Senya, K., Duah, A., Owusu-Ofori, A., Amugsi, J., Suglo, D., Bampoh, S. A., Hiebert, L., Njuguna, H., Ward, J. W., Plymoth, A., Roberts, L. R., Bockarie, A. S., Awuku, Y. A., & Obiri-Yeboah, D. (2022). A nationwide cross-sectional review of in-hospital hepatitis B virus testing and disease burden estimation in Ghana, 2016–2021. *BMC Public Health, 22*(1), 1–15.

National Center for Immunization Research & Surveillance. (2015). *Hepatitis B vaccines for Australians: NCIRS fact sheet*. Retrieved March 6, 2024, from https://ncirs.org.au/ncirs-fact-sheets-faqs/hepatitis-b-vaccines-for-australians

Ndunguru, B., Wilfred, D., Kapesa, A., Kilonzo, S. D., Mirambo, M., Hyera, F., & Massaga, F. (2023). Low uptake of hepatitis B vaccination among healthcare workers in primary health facilities in Mwanza region North-Western Tanzania. *Frontiers in Public Health, 11*(June), 1–9.

Obiri-Yeboah, D., Awuku, Y. A., Adjei, G., Cudjoe, O., Benjamin, A. H., Obboh, E., & Amoako-Sakyi, D. (2019). Post hepatitis B vaccination sero-conversion among health care workers in the Cape Coast Metropolis of Ghana. *PLoS ONE, 14*(6), 1–13.

Obirikorang, C., Opoku, S. K., Obirikorang, Y., Yorke, E. A. J., Donkoh, E. T., Chidera, C., Sarpong, D., Anto, E. O., Issahaku, R., Appeaning, M., Christian Nelson, E. N. B., Amakwah, B., Asamoah, E. A., Amoah, B., & Afraine, B. O. (2018). Awareness and occupational exposures to needlestick injuries among healthcare workers: A quantitative assessment in a Ghanaian metropolis. *Global Journal on Quality and Safety in Healthcare*, 4–5.https://doi.org/10.4103/JQSH.JQSH

Ofori-Asenso, R., & Agyeman, A. A. (2016). Hepatitis B in Ghana: A systematic review & meta-analysis of prevalence studies (1995–2015). *BMC Infectious Diseases, 16*(1), Article130.

Opiyo, N., & English, M. (2010). In-service training for health professionals to improve care of the seriously ill newborn or child in low and middle-income countries. *Cochrane Database Syst Rev, 4*(4). https://doi.org/10.1002/14651858.CD007071.pub2.In-service

Oppong, T. B., Amponsem-Boateng, C., Kyere, E. K. D., Wang, Y., Gheisari, Z., Oppong, E. E., Opolot, G., Duan, G., & Yang, H. (2020). Infection prevention and control preparedness level and associated determinants in 56 acute healthcare facilities in Ghana. *Infection and Drug Resistance, 13*, 4263–4271.

Osei, E., Niyilapah, J., Kofi Amenuvegbe, G., & Liu, Y. (2019). Hepatitis B knowledge, testing, and vaccination history among undergraduate public health students in Ghana. *BioMed Research International, 2019*. https://doi.org/10.1155/2019/7645106

Pan American Health Organization Regional Office. (2015). *Hepatitis B immunization of health workers: A comprehensive approach to the prevention of occupational transmission of blood-borne pathogens among health workers*. Retrieved from https://www.paho.org.dm.documents

Pappas, S. C., & Fisher, M. M. (1985). Preventing hepatitis B in health care workers. *Canadian Family Physician Medecin De Famille Canadien, 31*, 1941–1944.

Sagoe, C., & Pearson, R. (2001). Risks to healthcare workers in developing countries. *New England Journal of Medicine, 345*(7).

Senoo-Dogbey, V. E. (2021). Adherence to post exposure prophylaxis for Hepatitis B virus among health care workers in Accra , Ghana. *IOSR Journal of Nursing and Health Science (IOSR-JNHS), 10*(5), 52–59. https://doi.org/10.9790/1959-1005075259

Senoo-Dogbey, V. E. (2022). The knowledge of post-exposure prophylaxis for hepatitis B virus and related factors among health care workers in Accra Ghana. *Archives of Occupational Health, 6*(1), 1164–1170.

Senoo-Dogbey, V. E., Armah, D., & Wuaku, D. A. (2023a). Hepatitis B infection prevention: Audit of selected healthcare facilities in the Greater Accra Region, Ghana. *Infection Prevention in Practice, 5*(2), 100284. https://doi.org/10.1016/j.infpip.2023.100284

Senoo Dogbey, V. E., Armah, D., & Wuaku, A. D. (2023b). Hepatitis B virus vaccination post serological testing and antibody levels of vaccinated health care workers in Accra, Ghana. *Vaccine: X, 14*, 100294.

Senoo-Dogbey, V. E., & Wauku, D. A. (2022). Risk perception for Hepatitis B Virus (HBV) infection among health care workers in Accra, Ghana. *Clinical Epidemiology and Global Health, 18*, 101189.

Senoo-Dogbey, V. E., Wuaku, D. A., & Armah, D. (2023). Seroprevalence of Hepatitis B virus infection and associated factors among health care workers in Southern Ghana. *IJID Regions, 6*(November 2022), 84–89. https://doi.org/10.1016/j.ijregi.2023.01.009

Singhal, V., Bora, D., & Singh, S. (2009). Hepatitis B in health care workers: Indian scenario. *Journal of Laboratory Physicians, 1*(2), 41–48.

Suglo, R. E., Aku, F. Y., Anaman-Torgbor, J. A., & Tarkang, E. E. (2021). Predictors of adherence to HIV Post-Exposure Prophylaxis protocol among frontline healthcare workers at the Ho Teaching Hospital, Ghana. *International Journal of Infectious Diseases, 106*, 208–212.

Sunkwa-Mills, G., Senah, K., Breinholdt, M., Aberese-Ako, M., & Tersbøl, B. P. (2023). A qualitative study of infection prevention and control practices in the maternal units of two Ghanaian hospitals. *Antimicrobial Resistance and Infection Control, 12*(1), 1–15.

Świtalski, J., Wnuk, K., Tatara, T., Miazga, W., Wiśniewska, E., Banaś, T., Partyka, O., Karakiewicz-Krawczyk, K., Jurczak, J., Kaczmarski, M., Dykowska, G., Czerw, A., & Cipora, E. (2022). Interventions to increase patient safety in long-term care facilities—Umbrella review. *International Journal of Environmental Research and Public Health, 19*(22), 1–20.

Taneja, N., & Biswal, M. (2006). Safe disposal of infectious waste—Indian perspective. *Journal of Hospital Infection, 62*(4), 524–525.

Tawiah, P. A., Abaka-Yawson, A., Effah, E. S., Arhin-Wiredu, K., & Oppong, K. (2022). Prevalence and risk factors of hepatitis B virus infection among medical laboratory science students in a Ghanaian tertiary institution. *Journal of Health Research, 36*(3), 442–452.

Tiko, M. (2023). *Self-efficacy for Hepatitis B prevention among midwives*. In MPhil Thesis, University of Ghana.

Trepo, C., Chan, H., & Lok, A. (2014). Hepatitis B virus infection. *The Lancet, 384*(6), 2053–2063.

World Health Organization. (2019). *Minimum requirements for infection prevention and control programme*. World Health Organization.

World Health Organization. (2014). *Surveillance for vaccine preventable diseases*. World Health Organization.

Yassi, A., Lockhart, K., Sykes, M., Stime, B., & Spiegel, J. (2013). Effectiveness of joint health and safety committees: A realist review. *American Journal of Industrial Medicine, 56*(6), 424–438.

Zafar, A., Habib, F., Hadwani, R., Ejaz, M., Khowaja, K., Khowaja, R., & Irfan, S. (2009). Impact of infection control activities on the rate of needle stick injuries at a tertiary care hospital of Pakistan over a period of six years: An observational study. *BMC Infectious Diseases, 9*, 78. https://doi.org/10.1186/1471-2334-9-78

Zingg, W., Holmes, A., Dettenkofer, M., Goetting, T., Secci, F., Clack, L., Allegranzi, B., Magiorakos, A. P., Pittet, D., Carmeli, Y., Dittrich, A., Ebner, W., Edwards, R., Ferlie, E., Gastmeier, P., Hryniewicz, W., Kalenic, S., Kilpatrick, C., Sorknes, N., ... Vincent, C. (2015). Hospital organisation, management, and structure for prevention of health-care-associated infection: A systematic review and expert consensus. *The Lancet Infectious Diseases, 15*(2), 212–224.

CHAPTER 7

Health-in-all, Data Harmonisation, and Cross-sectoral Collaboration in Ghana's Health Sector

Alena Thiel

7.1 Introduction

Contemporary global health dynamics, especially novel diseases (e.g. Covid-19) and new environmental health concerns resulting from climate change, are putting additional pressure on already resource-scarce health systems in the Global South. Tackling these complex dynamics requires concerted efforts beyond the health system. As a response, Ghana's 2020 National Health Policy (NHP) promotes a whole-of-government and whole-of-society approach to delivering holistic, comprehensive, equitable, affordable, and responsive health services (NHP, 2020). This is in line with World Health Organization (WHO) and other multilateral health organisations, which have for some time promoted "Health in All Policies" (HiAP). HiAP "recognizes that population health is not merely

A. Thiel (✉)
Martin-Luther-University Halle-Wittenberg, Halle, Germany
e-mail: alena.thiel@ethnologie.uni-halle.de

A. Thiel and S. A. Ntewusu (eds.), *The Social Life of Health Data*,
https://doi.org/10.1007/978-981-97-3500-6_7

a product of health sector programmes but largely determined by policies that guide actions beyond the health sector. Policy in every sector of government can potentially affect health and inequities in health" (WHO, n.d.). At the same time, agendas such as "one-health" equally demand a "collaborative, multisectoral, and transdisciplinary approach—working at the local, regional, national, and global levels—with the goal of achieving optimal health outcomes recognizing the interconnection between people, animals, plants, and their shared environment" (CDC, 2023).

While the goal of one-health and health-in-all seems to be on everybody's lips in policy, development, and academic circles, the digital infrastructures required for these agendas remain surprisingly vague. Yet cross-sectoral health interventions, e.g. in public health emergencies, require specific work in data harmonisation and sharing across institutional boundaries. This chapter rearticulates the by now well-established observation that database innovations affect both material devices, software, and forms of expertise, but also the organisation of personnel, resources, and ideas associated with them. This is equally true for the datafication of health, which "is as much, and maybe more, about aligning organisational-political actors as it is about technical solutions" (Sæbo et al., 2011, p. 42). In view of this, the chapter sets out to discuss the infrastructural arrangements underlying the production and cross-sector circulation of health data in Ghana. Centrally, the chapter traces the Ghanaian health system's investments in data standards, but also the specific adaptations that emerge from them, as well as the (unintended) consequences of digital innovations for health practitioners' routine data practices. Pointing to the work of standard case definitions, epidemiological thresholds, plotted graphs, and informal reporting channels, among other types of knowledge technologies, the chapter illustrates the complex collaboration of digital tools and their adaptations in Ghanaian health data practices.

Standardisation here is understood with reference to the now classic work by Bowker and Star (1999) on this issue. Because of its facilitating role in coordinating distributed work and cognition, standardisation is the precondition for the operation of any working infrastructure (Bowker & Star, 1999, p. 325, see also Lampland & Star, 2008). In digital systems in particular, classifications and the standards they enable are ubiquitous. As standards are applied at increasing scale, they converge and get locked into material technology as well as immaterial forms of organisation, and hence become part of "ever more densely interconnected" and increasingly irreversible large-scale information systems (Bowker & Star, 1999, pp. 135, 326). Yet, despite their immersion into the background of information systems, standards exert a significant structuring, or regulatory force, over our lives—at times to unintended material effect (see Bowker & Star, 1999 on the issue of "torque"). In view of these reflections, this chapter follows the call to understand standardisation processes as simultaneously material and symbolic, a "juncture of social organization, moral order, and layers of technical integration," and which always require significant translation into local sites (Bowker & Star, 1999, p. 33, see also Lampland & Star, 2008).

The chapter unfolds by first giving a brief overview of the evolution of (digital) health records in Ghana. It then discusses the setup of digital health registration and the potential for intersectoral interoperability in moments of public health emergencies. Data for this chapter was collected as part of the project "How Democracies Know" (DFG TH2432/2–1) at the Martin-Luther-University Halle-Wittenberg. Ethnographic fieldwork was carried out with district, regional, and national-level health information managers in the Greater Accra, Upper West, and Bono East regions. In addition to face-to-face interviews and narrative "walk-throughs" of relevant computational systems and interfaces (Light et al., 2018; Troeger & Bock, 2022), interviews were conducted remotely during the Covid-19 pandemic to address the risk of infection, and to adhere to ethical and public health guidelines defined by the Ghana Health Service Research Ethics Committee. Motivated by the still under-represented perspective of the digital labour required to maintain the functionality of digital health information systems (Star & Strauss, 1999), the data collection focused on mid-level data managers as the key experts in aggregating health data at district, regional, and national levels, and at connecting across institutional boundaries.

7.2 The Evolution of (digital) Health in Ghana

Ghana's healthcare system dates back to colonial times, when a system modelled on the British colonial power provided only marginal care for those unable to pay out of pocket (Abebrese, 2011, see also Chapters 2 and 3 in this edition on the changing rationales of public health interventions). Although independence in 1957 brought with it a brief period of free and universal health care, following the 1966 coup d'état against independence leader Kwame Nkrumah, various fees were gradually introduced, which eventually reduced health care to a direct payment, or "cash-and-carry" healthcare system (Carbone, 2011). With the country's multiparty opening of 1992 and the return to democracy following decades of political unrest, health care again became a central political issue in the 1990s. In 1996, a sector-wide approach to health policy was adopted, and in 1997, a Health Fund was launched in which development partners pooled resources for the expansion of mutual health organisations. However, as these arrangements covered only about 1% of the population, they raised concerns about the equity of the system's central funding, and hence remained highly contested (Carbone, 2011, p. 398; Sulzbach et al., 2005). In 2003, a contributory health insurance scheme was therefore introduced, which marked the first step towards broader health coverage (Carbone, 2011, p. 394). In 2012, the district-based organisational structure of the National Health Insurance Scheme was reformed into today's centralised system, making the Ghanaian health system available to increasingly large parts of the population, and providing free health care for children and recipients of Ghana's LEAP poverty alleviation programme (Abebrese, 2011, p. 28; Grebe, 2015, pp. 20, 23).

A central component of the commitment of Ghana's health system towards universal health care relates to the digitisation of health records. The call for integrated data warehousing, and the standardising and integrating of health data, first emerged from international organisations towards the end of the 2000s. Data warehouses, according to the official rationale, organise data from partly overlapping subsystems run by different vertical health programmes into one central database framework (Sæbo et al., 2011). This represented a significant challenge for the Ghanaian health information system of the early 2000s. Data production was fragmented, and data use remained limited to local facilities and districts (Adaletey et al., 2013, p. 11). Although routine health records were the main source of information for health managers at the district level, most data managers relied "on paper form of storage as the only means of storing data and information" (Boadu, 2004, n.p.). Therefore, transforming the raw data into the required information was extremely labour-intensive, and "decisions based on personal intuition" remained the norm (ibid.). Where data was centralised, "little feedback [was] given back to the periphery," which "contributed to an inefficient, irrelevant and redundant HIS [health information system]" (Adaletey et al., 2013,

p. 11, see also Odei-Lartey et al., 2020, p. 515) in which information was solely disseminated through meetings, circulars, and reports, and decisions were therefore frequently delayed (Boadu, 2004, n.p.).

In view of these problems, in 2007 the District Health Information Management System (DHIMS) was rolled out with support from the European Union. The system not only failed to meet demands, but was further described as negatively affecting healthcare delivery, as it forced stakeholders to "develop parallel reporting systems to enable them to meet data demands of their sponsors," while few users could access and benefit from the system, and automation of reporting and analysis remained limited (Adaletey et al., 2013, p. 12). As a response, in 2012 Ghana updated its HIS to DHIMS2, based on the widely used DHIS2 software (District Health Information System). DHIS2 is a free, open-source software developed at the University of Oslo for the purpose of data collection on healthcare provision, and the integration of data warehouses for essential health data, but also for the management of processes related to information sharing, analysis, and dissemination. More recently, DHIS2 has provided tools for emergency responses to the Covid-19 pandemic and the subsequent vaccination roll-out, but also addresses emerging issues such as environmental health concerns (DHIS2, n.d.). Updating to DHIS2 significantly altered the information flow in Ghana's HIS. Most importantly, according to the planners, issues of data silos and duplication were addressed, which according to the policymakers provided the basis for a more democratic data production and analysis for all users of the system (Adaletey et al., 2013, p. 12, see also Jolliffe et al., 2015). One informant confirmed this at the district level: "In what we are doing here, we are implementing the national standard of DHIMS2."[1] And pointing to the importance of the system for data quality assurance, he added: "Before then, (…) we had too many errors, so we needed access at our level to correct the data." District-level data managers emphasise that being able to review the data at the district or municipal level allows direct feedback to defaulting facilities, and targeted training of staff tasked with data entry, where errors occur most frequently.

These observations point us to the labour of standardising health data, from implementing the roll-out of a digital health information management system to the training and supervision of staff for data entry. Yet

[1] Interview, GHS, UWR, 2023.

while significant scholarly attention has been expended on DHIS2, e.g. in the software developers' annual DHIS2 conference and online community of practice, as well as from several Ghanaian and international scholars writing about the system's design (Adaletey et al., 2013; Miscione, 2008; Odei-Lartey et al., 2020; Ofosu, 2012; Sæbo et al., 2011), there is still a need for the critical interrogation of how DHIMS2 restructures digital labour in Ghana's health sector. The subsequent sections aim to respond to this need.

7.3 Database Access and the Labour of Digital Health

DHIMS2 records service provision of all health facilities across the territory of Ghana, and thereby provides the basis for quantifying myriad health indicators for planning and intervention. Streamlining data production in this context requires the participation of several types of staff and devices. By design, DHIMS2 is populated "through use": that is, the idea is for community health workers (CHW) to use the system's mobile e-tracker application to keep patients' records up to date. However, planners note, nation-wide implementation of the tracker app remains limited due to lack of hardware. Besides population of the database through use, data is further entered into DHIMS2 through monthly routine tallies of reported services by all health facilities (Odei-Lartey et al., 2020, p. 516; Ofosu, 2012, p. 9). From the central data managers' point of view, the task of data entry is necessarily a joint effort. "We have the community, the sub-district, district, and municipal, and regional levels of data entry. The community level is at the health facilities, CHPS[2] compounds, and then some private clinics. The sub-district is at the level of the health centres. And then we have the regional and district hospitals."[3] At the community level, health records are put together by CHWs, and are then reviewed by a supervising health professional, before a "reporting form is

[2] A CHPS compound, or National Community and Health Planning and Services compound, provides health services in close proximity to the community to reduce geographical access barriers (Awoonor-Williams et al., n.d.). Community nurses provide home visits to monitor maternal and child health and provide childhood vaccinations, among many other public health interventions, e.g. community sensitisation in the context of the Covid-19 pandemic.

[3] Interview, GHS, Bono East, 2023.

generated for review by the 'district data validation team' which keys the data into the DHIMS2 application" (Kwame Adu, 2014, p. 5). At the regional level, another validation team checks the data and "signs it off for its use at the national level" (Kwame Adu, 2014, p. 6).

As a platform, DHIS2 formats data production in two moments: first, the moment of data capture, and second, the reporting stage. Based on the district-wide aggregation of health records, periodic report statements are compiled which track indicators. These indicators include per capita attendance of facilities defined by age groups and by insurance method, caseload, and crucially, the incidence and prevalence of about 100 priority diseases.[4] Reporting and visualisation then proceed along pre-programmed data-set reports, pivot tables, and layered map-outs of key indicators at the level of Ghana's health districts. DHIS2 then automatically generates indicators and displays them according to the user's configurations of the system's dashboard.

Moving beyond the default design of DHIS2 as a platform, and exploring practices of data entry into DHIMS2, reveals a more nuanced picture of the digital labour required for sustaining the system, and allows an exploration of the labour involved in populating DHIMS2.

DHIMS2 not only streamlines formats, but also temporalities of data production. In the case of Ghana's digital health register, this district-level health information manager described the process of data entry as highly complex, especially so in the interest of assuring synchronicity and continuous data quality:

> We do data entry in a particular timeline. From 1st to 5th of every month the reports come from sub-districts to our offices, the officers here have the capacity to vet and correct errors made, such as pregnancy in males, or errors such as 1 and 1 adds to 3. Then we prompt the facility [to correct mistakes]. We also keep our logbook for all received reports. We list all reports that we are supposed to receive. The log indicates submission date and errors we identified. We use these for capacity training, for example we find that there are lots of errors in the reports of midwives. So, we can direct our training there. It also allows us to measure timeliness. And we can compare against the copies in the facilities, so if one is missing, we can

[4] These diseases are regularly monitored by the Ghana Health Service (GHS), along with close observation of increases in the "other" category, which allows monitoring of (new) diseases of specific concern, and periodically lumps them into new categories of emerging conditions, such as in recent years Covid-19, H1N1, or Ebola.

> reconcile it. (...) From 5th to 10th of each month, we set our own target to enter all data [into DHIMS2]. Nationally, the data is due at the 15th but because sometimes you make a mistake, this allows us to still correct something after data validation. (interview, GHS, UWR, 2023)

Strauss and Star (1999) refer to the invisible "backstage" labour of infrastructuring when they foreground the work of tinkering and adjusting that sustains (data) infrastructures' operations. Because reporting templates structure everything from how the data is generated at the point of the outpatient department record (OPD record), to how it is summarised and tallied at decentral level, and transmitted nationally through DHIMS2, significant backstage labour goes into capacity training to ensure this level of standardisation. As this data manager explained: "Some of the data we enter at the [district] office. Especially clinical data, morbidity, and malaria. But we are building the capacity for health staff to enter it themselves" at the facilities. "The nature of the training is very practical, first you get an overview of DHIMS, its functionalities, reporting formats for data entry. Once you are trained, we just monitor you." This, the data manager argues further, enhances ownership and therefore also data quality. "The reason we want the health staff [to do the data entry] is ownership. Once you have access you can extract [what you need in your work]. Based on monthly reporting you will see where the cases are coming from. We are channelling health information to where it is generated, and that adds to its quality," because data producers also become users of the data.[5]

Given the capacity-building aspect of DHIMS2, selection for training is presented as a privilege. "The sequence is that we train you, then you will get an account [with DHIMS2] and then you receive clearance. The fellowship selection entails that you are IT inclined, using computer, tablets. You have to have appreciation for our reporting format, so you have to have worked with health data already. You need to be committed to the work, not going here today, there tomorrow...but be available to apply it."[6] In other words, the investment in training requires significant resources which should benefit the health system in the long term.

In contrast to these data managers' depiction of capacity building, scholars have pointed to the ambiguous effects of datafying health on

[5] Interview, GHS, UWR, 2023.

[6] Ibid.

the surveillance of health staff and the expansion of neoliberal accounting logics (Al Dahdah, 2015). These ideas are confirmed in my interviews with national-level policy planners, who note: "If you do not report in DHIS2 it means the service is not provided and we do not pay you."[7] At the same time, when speaking to community health workers, datafication did not appear to relay crucial information on community health back to inform their work, hence challenging the discourse of ownership and raising questions about the burden of datafication and the location of its generative effects.

Moreover, as noted above, lack of hardware limits the potential of the technology's design. "So very useful these days is the e-tracker, which is something like an electronic register. [...] The hard copies, you keep them, but electronic registers you can extract immediately. When you travel you have all files with you." Yet, this district-level data manager admitted, "the only challenge is to provide the devices."[8] This account points us to the complexity of the assemblage of trained staff, functioning devices, and network capacity, among many other elements, that are needed to ensure the efficiency gains promised in the course of health system digitalisation, but also the constant tension between infrastructure's realities (e.g. absent or broken devices) and its implicit assumptions (e.g. that health staff will populate the HIS with data "through use").

Such tensions become articulated at various moments. As this data manager points out,[9] another limiting factor within DHIMS2 is that there is "so much data on the system and a lot of people are hooked on the server, it slows down." For this professional, the obvious solution is to "expand the workspace," especially in the interest of securing historical data. Yet his experience is very different. "For managing the space, they take off the historical data. If you do not have your own backup, you cannot access it [any longer]." From the point of view of local planners, this is highly problematic, as public health officials routinely rely on past health records to predict seasonal disease trends. Such tensions, this informant explained further, are a symptom of a larger geopolitical issue. "The hosting of DHIMS is not in Ghana. As a health service [GHS] should get our own server. For ownership of the data. You don't have absolute

[7] Interview, MOH, Accra, 2021.

[8] Interview, GHS, UWR, 2023.

[9] Ibid.

control over your data." This last statement points directly at the structuring force of standardisation, and its immersion in relations of power. The limitations listed here are in no way aimed at minimising the crucially important role of standards in promoting evidence-based decisions and accelerating life-saving interventions. Nonetheless, it serves as a reminder that standards do not usually operate without friction, and the labour required to even out tensions (while being necessarily black-boxed in the standard itself) deserves recognition. The next section provides further illustrations of the significance of standards in processes of monitoring health for targeted health planning and expenditure.

7.4 Monitoring and the Standardisation of Health Indicators

The production of routine health data is of crucial importance for the planning, organisation, and delivery of health services at the level of management (e.g. for the definition of health indicators), but it requires significant investments in regulation, material technologies and immaterial forms of organisation, as well as creative adaptations to translate and fit into local contexts of use. Some thoughts have already been expressed on the labour required to populate the health register. Yet the Ghanaian health data infrastructure itself also involves significant work to achieve standardisation.

Data production is standardised, first, through regular vetting of health facilities by the Health Facilities Regulatory Authority (HeFRA), which ties operational licenses to compliance with reporting in DHIMS2. While routine reporting through standardised templates has been widely rolled out, some institutions that existed prior to the Health Institutions and Facilities Act, 2011 (Act 829) have not fully been on-boarded onto DHIMS2, thus requiring further efforts to secure country-wide implementation. Beyond this aspect of licensing, DHIMS2 itself has to be continuously maintained and updated. For this purpose, GHS runs the Centre for Health Information Management (CHIM) under its Information, Monitoring, and Evaluation Department for ensuring the technical harmonisation of health data production. According to its mandate, CHIM is responsible for "collating, analyzing and storing all data on service utilization" nation-wide, but also to "organize reporting systems, initiate mechanisms that ensure data reliability and reflect the true level of health performance," and for "leading and strengthening data and information support, training in data management and providing assistance in data management within other divisions" (GHS, 2023).

Finally, the very indicators produced through digital quantification do not exist in isolation from the political, organisational, and technological contexts of their production. According to a representative at the Ministry of Health, three major groups in the health sector define how indicators are produced for the purpose of monitoring the Ghanaian health sector. First, the interagency leadership committee, chaired by the Minister of Health, brings together all heads of agencies (the FDA, GHS, Ambulance Service, among others). Second, the national technical quality committee guides the implementation of the national health strategy. And third, the health sector working group, which is a wider group of technical experts, the development partners, and CSOs as the mouthpiece of the communities, collectively reviews the progress made in health indicators. This third group meets every four years to define the health sector medium-term development plan and deliver an Aid Memoir during the Health Summit, in which goals are set, progress is evaluated, and multisectoral activities are aligned along the SDGs. Additionally, Ghana's donor-oriented health programmes, e.g. the National Malaria Control Programme, are subject to internationally standardised tools for monitoring and evaluation.

In this assemblage, DHIMS2's core function is to provide routine and timely reviews of the performance of the health system in a comparable manner. This means that, while selected indicators are generated right away for use in the district or municipality and are reported directly to the Director of the Health Directorate, they ultimately serve to compare trends in each location.[10]

Standard reporting formats render health sector performance comparable across districts, enabling quarterly, half-yearly, and annual reviews. "We compare performance of facility, sub-district and also with other districts. We organise fora for review where all meet to present and discuss developments. We then come out with reasons why we are doing well,

[10] "We have direct targets we set for ourselves, for example the maternal mortality ratio." Any of these indicators of special attention differ by region. For example, in the three northern regions, due to similar socio-economic concerns, public health officials "give extra eye to meningitis," while also monitoring maternal and child mortality, and anaemia in pregnancy. Moreover, DHIMS2 helps health officials to "still keep tracks on Covid-19 in line with international demand" (interview, GHS, UWR, 2023).

what are interventions that worked or didn't work. If sub-districts are doing well, we ask them to share what they have done and share with others at the regional level." These fora include what this planner refers to as "partners" from the Nursing and Midwifery Council, NGOs, the District Assembly, Ambulance Service, Ghana Police, private health facilities, and local health committees including chiefs and elders, but also representatives from national-level institutions, along with the media and other stakeholders. "They come to give their input to share ideas and report on performance, but also the challenges we face as a service to handle, so we ask our partners for help and give timelines for action."[11]

Data collection at the district level, in other words, represents an important moment of synchronisation, which brings health data into cross-sectoral dialogue. Standardisation here provides an important vector of "comparity" (Schinkel 2016) across regionally diverse health issues. At the local planning level, specific indicators are grouped under the health sector's centrally defined key objectives. Specifically, at the time of the study, Ghana's Health Sector Medium Term Development Plan (2018–2022) defined the national health objectives as follows:

1. Ensure sustainable, affordable, equitable, and easily accessible healthcare service;
2. Reduce morbidity and mortality, and intensify prevention and control of noncommunicable diseases;
3. Enhance efficiency in governance and management; and
4. Intensify prevention and control of communicable diseases.

A range of specific sector indicators is then grouped under these four objectives, including for example, maternal mortality, the percentage of pregnant women who are anaemic at 36 weeks, vitamin A coverage, Penta-3 coverage, the institutional maternal mortality rate, U5 malaria, family planning acceptance weeks, long-term couple year protection, percentage of skilled deliveries, postnatal care seen within 40 hours, the proportion of children given insecticide-treated bed nets, measles and rubella vaccinations, and patronage of service (OPD per capita), among myriad other indicators. The production of these performance indicators as a key output of DHIMS2 is also relevant far beyond the annual holistic

[11] Interview, GHS, UWR, 2023.

assessment. Displayed on large posters in the district offices, colour-coded areas were earmarked for intervention and informed comparative, cross-district attention in public health planning, and monitoring all year round.

Beyond datafication at the district level, DHIMS2 data further provides the ground for health sector's holistic assessment at national scale. Once aggregated at the national headquarters of GHS, the standardised reporting of all districts and municipalities is collated and presented at the annual Health Summit organised by Ghana's Ministry of Health. At the national level, the Holistic Assessment tool pools DHIMS2 data together with data produced by the Health Facility Regulatory Agency (HeFRA), the Food and Drugs Authority (FDA), and the health sector regulatory agencies (the Pharmacy Council, Alternative Medicine Authority, morgues and mortuaries, Ambulance Service, and Blood Bank). Based on data provided by these bodies, key processes and holistic indicators are calculated at the Ministry of Health during the annual inter-agency review meetings, as well as at the moment of peer-review in service delivery between facilities—all in the interest of streamlining collaboration and setting the health policy for the years to come.

In the remainder of the chapter, I will build on these insights to discuss the role of health data infrastructure in intersectoral health interventions. Specifically, the following section details the forms of organisation (of digital and analogue technologies, as well as various forms of expertise) required to implement intersectoral data-sharing in contexts of public health emergencies, where such collaboration is most critical for timely intervention and the containment of outbreaks.

7.5 Standardisation and the Problem of Cross-sectoral Intervention

According to my interlocutors, standardisation in health data is aimed at harmonising and de-duplicating information flows in health care "so that one agency's output becomes another's input."[12] As defined by the NHP (2020), Ghana's Ministry of Health promotes multisectoral action, and seeks to "engage relevant stakeholders including local communities to strengthen health care decisions and responsibility" while also seeking

[12] Interview, MOH, Accra, 2021.

to "address (broader) economic, social and environmental determinants and risk factors" in health. Involving "more stakeholders in the achievement of Health for All," as per the official rationale, is crucial to address conflicts of interest, and to promote transparency and participatory governance (NHP, 2020). Moreover, according to the NHP, while "Ghana has over the years, established discrete programmes in response to specific health and disease problems, such as Malaria, TB, HIV/AIDS, maternal and child health, and NCDs (...) the challenge remains to ensure that these programmes are fully integrated as a package" (ibid.). Ghana's 2020 NHP further "recognizes that the disease burden and its impact on segments of the population is influenced by the national demographics, geographical distribution and the socio-economic status of the population." Consequently, targeting interventions to where they are most needed requires detailed knowledge and hence cross-sectoral data sharing about the population, to be able to appropriately design services and account for populations with unique needs (ibid.).

Yet, to date, cross-sectoral data sharing between national-level government organisations occurs mainly through informal avenues, such as personal communication, staff exchanges, or ad-hoc data requests, oftentimes involving requests for payment for specific datasets.[13] Data-sharing between organisations thus remains the exception rather than the norm. This section looks at one such exception, namely the collaboration of emergency agencies in moments of localised[14] public health crises.

7.5.1 *Infrastructures of Disease Control*

Public health emergencies require concerted action across institutional boundaries. This section takes such an emergency, the case of cerebrospinal meningitis, as a case to explore how digital tools facilitate collaboration across public sector agencies. Before proceeding, it is necessary to understand the information collected for the purpose of controlling meningitis outbreaks.

[13] Interview, CHIM, Accra, 2021.

[14] In such sites, "turf wars" between centralised institutions are limited by mutual dependencies (cf. Thiel 2020), the localised focus on specific issues mobilises engagement, and communication channels function relatively unconstrained by bureaucratic formatting.

Meningitis outbreaks are seasonal events that mainly occur in Ghana's dry season, starting from November each year. Due to this seasonal characteristic, public health officials are habituated to anticipate outbreaks of meningitis at specific times of the year, which not least also manifests in their routine data practices. For example, disease control officers direct their ongoing data collections and retrospective analyses of historical health records to identify distinct (spatial and temporal) patterns of disease spread between specific localities and vocational groups, along with weather and vegetation patterns impacting these dynamics.

Disease Control Units (DCUs) are institutionally anchored in Ghana's district-based health directorates, and are tasked with the prevention and control of disease through public health interventions. Besides meningitis, they are concerned with all diseases pertinent to public health, including malaria, tuberculosis, HIV, neglected tropical diseases, emerging and re-emerging diseases, as well as any events of public health concern, such as snake bites. While the clinical work of disease control occurs in the health facilities, the DCU is responsible for "all the administrative components," including data work, and the management of processes. Specifically, the DCU identifies officers at all facilities, and trains these liaisons "at all levels, both the hospital level (i.e. regional) and the CHPS zone" to respond to emerging and re-emerging diseases.[15] Across these different scales, DCUs set the priority of their attention, "that is we rank the facilities by high to low priority. If you have high OPD attendance there is a high likeliness of recording cases, especially if you have OPD over 100.000. Our medium priority are the health centres, which might not even detain clients, the 'treat and go facilities'...Based on this prioritization we carry out our daily, weekly and monthly reviews" where high priority facilities are reviewed daily, and lower priority facilities less frequently.[16]

When this DCU officer refers to periodic "reviews," this entails the revision of health records at the facility by officers trained by the DCU. "As municipality, we have a team of surveillance officers who are trained in data collection and [who] in turn train their staff at the hospital and health centre level."[17] This entails, first, the sensitisation of clinicians to

[15] Interview, DCU, UWR, 2023.

[16] Ibid.

[17] Ibid.

update their knowledge of the WHO standard case definitions, in order to detect cases. When a clinician suspects a case at the facility level using the standard case definition, this case is reported through the OPD register, capturing biodata, age, address, diagnosis, and later confirmed diagnosis. Simultaneously, the clinician contacts the Disease Control Officer at the facility to come in and carry out the record review. The officer will review all records for the period, and look for cases the clinician might have overlooked. “So, in addition to fever, they may be looking for stiff neck, unconsciousness as signs of meningitis. Based on the review, they may bring in the patient again to follow up. Maybe someone presented with a fever but was not diagnosed as such.” It is the duty of the officer to ensure the suspected patient is treated and samples are taken to confirm the suspicion, by lumbar puncture in the case of meningitis. Then the case-based form is filled with basic information about the initial diagnosis, after which it is sent to the laboratory for confirmation. From there the case-based form is brought from the facility to the municipal office for line listing, that is to say populating a running sheet with all the cases.

> Immediately when we receive them, the paper copies of the case-based investigation forms are entered into SORMAS and [this] is immediately transmitted to Accra. This is our first point of data collection already. We have our line lists, we enter into SORMAS, where we can also pull the data locally to use for decision making. (interview, DCU, UWR, 2023)

Like DHIS2, the Surveillance Outbreak Response Management & Analysis System (SORMAS) is an open-source software that operates alongside DHIMS2 to facilitate the early detection of infections and the management of epidemics. SORMAS provides the software infrastructure for hospitals, laboratories, and public health officers, among others, to collaborate in the fight against the spread of disease. In Ghana, SORMAS runs on designated tablets provided by GHS with servers located at the Ghana Revenue Authority and data owned and controlled by GHS Disease Surveillance at the GHS HQ in Accra. Similar to DHIMS2, SORMAS creates differential data access. “At higher level, they can see graphs and the like [to compare trends and locations]. We have limited analyses, we see the cases, percentages, whether all data is complete at our end,” this DCU officer at the district level explained.[18]

[18] Ibid.

In addition to SORMAS, confirmed cases are then also entered into DHIS2's communicable disease form 1 (CD1), which collects all the data from the facility level right to the municipality. But, as this DCU officer explains, "at our level, our way of tracking is the line listing. So, if SORMAS fails, we should be able to trace all diseases of public health importance."[19] The DCU then monitors whether there is an outbreak or not by looking at defined thresholds. Pointing at a centrally located graph and table at the wall next to his desk, this DCU officer explains: "We first have an alert at 3 cases per 100.000, at 10 per 100.000 we have an epidemic. So, we monitor per week, with cases on the left [y-axis] and the week to the right [x-axis]. At the alert level we start preparing for a possible epidemic. But we need to look beyond the numbers. At the level of the CHPS zone, if the community is small, 1 case is already an epidemic. Especially if the population is less than 30.000."

The last statement begins to illustrate how standardisation is never absolute. My informants in fact attest to various adjustments that are made in local contexts. "In 2022, there were cases in the municipality. And we observed a doubling effect. So now, if we see that there are twice the number of cases than what we saw last year, we consider it an epidemic irrespective of the [other] parameters."[20] And in relation to the standard case definitions, this same team explains, some localities in the North of Ghana experience cases of meningitis that differ in their symptoms.

> We tell them to be mindful with the standard case definitions. The definition [for meningitis] is symptoms of fever, but we expand to presenting with a history of fever. Our people before they see the doctor, they may buy medication so when they are seen they may not present with fever. But they may be the epidemiological link in case of an outbreak. The standard has to be maintained, but you need to make adjustments. Based on cultural beliefs, what people do. Or [in a distinct locality], there we have a lot of meningitis cases that present differently. We need to review locally what the standard case definition entails to include other symptoms [and] adjust our instruments to this.

DCU officers also adapt their specific data practices to this end. Besides the standard line lists, this officer explains,

[19] Ibid.

[20] Ibid.

> we also use the spot map. So, we see that there is something going on there. The case-based forms contain personal info, lab report and other information like immunisations. This includes their biodata, geographical location, medical history, laboratory, and final outcome. (…) At our level, we would want to know who are those who are affected? The time factor is very important. And the place. We use [the spot map] to go where the cases are coming from, like particular parts of town. So, we can target our intervention and know where to divert our little resources.[21]

DCU officers further explained to me the importance of their accumulated experience in local sites, or a certain attunement to the types of connections that become visible in their mapping, e.g. based on mobility patterns associated with certain economic activities such as farming, that cannot be contained in line lists but nonetheless structure the attention of the public health experts. "It is essential, so next we have 500 cases we know based on our present numbers how to estimate cases and interventions, based on our knowledge of how groups of the population, like farmers, have contact," and how the disease will behave in this context.

Especially in remote contexts, reporting is further subject to potential time lags as health officials need to travel long distances to reach each facility. "What we enter into DHIMS platform is based on the hard copies they bring [from the facilities]. In there, we collate all diseases and cases of maternal mortality. Therefore, we need (…) digital tools. Our furthest facility is one day of travel away from here. If they transmit the info digitally, by the time they transmit the records," any intervention will inevitably be late.[22] To counteract such delays and accelerate reporting, DCUs across Ghana use alternative channels, such as WhatsApp groups. "We have all sub-municipalities put in [WhatsApp] groups. The data is sent right from the facilities. All cases reported through here are entered into SORMAS within 2–3 hours. (…) On the national level they also have this for the sixteen regions. This is our 'no bureaucracy mode of reporting.' So, by 12 o'clock, everything has reached the national level."[23] Using openly available software that runs on any smartphone or tablet, this mode of communication seems to at least partly contradict the logic of standardised interfaces for channelling information

[21] Ibid.

[22] Ibid.

[23] Ibid.

flows. Yet, also here DCU officers enforce a strict reporting standard,[24] and as a result DCU officers can effortlessly draw up any information from the groups in a matter of seconds.

7.5.2 *Inter-agency Collaboration in Public Health Emergencies*

Standardisation and adaptability prepare DCUs to respond to public health emergencies, but they are also central for interagency collaboration. Once there is an epidemic as defined by a certain threshold (10/100,000 for the case of meningitis), there arises the need of scaling up capacity. From the perspective of the DCU, this means that "you also need more resources, [hence] we activate the rapid response team [RRT] and the public health emergency management committee."

The RRT consists of technical personnel that can manage known cases, and that ensure the reporting of new ones. In the facilities, there are medical doctors, the lab, nurses, and pharmacists. "We draw them together through the [facilities'] heads to do the extra work, review the literature and refresh their knowledge." The public health emergency committee, in contrast, is located at the district office. It comprises the District and Municipal Chief Executives, a representative of the Ghana Education Service who assists in public health campaigns in the schools, as well as representatives from the Directorate of Agriculture and the National Disaster Management Organisation (NADMO). Representatives from the security services support the committee by enacting bylaws, e.g. to police a lock-down or quarantine. "We also ask the police to escort when we go there at night. The ambulance services, when they move in congested areas, the police helps." The traditional rulers, religious bodies, and other groups may also be invited if their support is deemed necessary. Moreover, "the RRTs are also members [of the committee]. They do most of the reporting work. The committee meets and reviews the cases and decides on how to control the outbreak, implement and monitor. They decide to mobilize resources, for example to sponsor free treatment, we need the political heads to clear the budget."[25]

[24] For each facility, clearly saved under its name in the respective group, a list of three to four types of events was reported, along with its frequencies, in a standard format, e.g. "snake bite: 3."

[25] Interview, GHS, UWR, 2023.

These interactions follow clearly defined structures laid out in annual epidemic preparedness plans that contain all the protocols to contain meningitis. Centrally, the plan provides the procedure in case of an outbreak and identifies the RRT members, "because in an outbreak you do not want people to ask who is responsible."[26] The plan's terms of reference also define what the committee members are supposed to do, and the essential commodities needed for outbreak control and management. "So you can see whether you have everything you need. What is the budget? What are the essential medications? You calculate the amount you need in the pharmacies and labs," but also "the operational dimension. The document you are going to use," and any other dimension of budgeting and planning.

The case of public health emergencies shows that cross-sectoral collaboration is a matter of effectively communicating the needs and contributions of specific agencies. "For example, with anthrax, we need personnel of MOFA [Ministry of Food and Agriculture] to vaccinate the cattle."[27] In these moments, my informants report, digital and analogue infrastructures are creatively layered onto each other. Paper-based preparedness plans identify lines of command, while DHIMS2 plays a central role as well. For zoonotic diseases for example, "DHIMS connects us to Veterinary Service. If there is any zoonotic disease they will be invited to follow up."[28] As was mentioned above, due to time constraints, cross-sectoral requests for data in this arrangement, are routinely channelled through the committees' WhatsApp channels.

This technical choice, a DCU officer mentioned, requires some sense of care, as the records of the collaborating agencies do not necessarily correspond with what will be shared. "Whatever veterinary is capturing [in their system] it will not reach us. ... Now if you go into their system, it is different from what we see here [in the WhatsApp channel]." These observations indicate that Health-in-All and One-Health agendas are present in Ghana's health policy circles and inform inter-agency collaborations, especially in public health emergencies. Infrastructurally, however, data-sharing agreements and platforms remain largely informal, and although public health professionals enforce particular standards,

[26] Ibid.

[27] Interview, GHS, Bono East, 2023.

[28] Ibid.

they also point to the limited capacity for data quality assurance and monitoring.

To achieve inter-sectoral collaboration, local staff of Ghana Health Service (GHS) and other members of the district-level emergency committee mobilise "decentral interoperability." The coordinating function of decentral sites of data production in Ghana's district-based emergency committees can hardly be overstated. While national-level disaster organisations only share limited information, district emergency committees integrate and coordinate information on disasters horizontally across institutional boundaries, and crucially distribute early warning information vertically to regional and national decision-makers. They manage to do this, one MCE in my study laid out, but maintaining short communication lines, personal knowledge, and crucially, the skillful combination of these analogue channels with the adaptation of standard and non-standard digital tools for accelerating data sharing.

7.6 Conclusion

This chapter set out to discuss the infrastructural arrangements underlying the production and circulation of health data in Ghana. In addition to promoting efficiency, transparency, and accountability in health care, the digitisation of the Ghanaian health register has in recent years come to align with the larger promise of interoperable population data systems, and the routine analysis of administrative health records. This is a trend that will undoubtedly develop in the future. Asked about their techno-optimist orientations, this policy planner detailed: "My vision is to have electronic patient records. We are currently reviewing our referral policy in order to move towards electronic referrals. So, once I do the referral, I can follow up and get electronic feedback. This is to have a more holistic way of collecting and sharing data, of course being mindful of the Data Protection Act."[29] In a related (neoliberal) logic, communities and individuals are envisioned to become part of the data production process. "The patient has to become more responsible for their own health (...) they need tools to self-observe."[30]

[29] Interview, MOH, Accra, 2021.

[30] Ibid.

However, my observations problematise the claim that digitalisation undoubtedly facilitates better care practices. Data practices, I have shown, are fundamentally geared at logics of monitoring and accountability. Since global health contexts have formatted care in terms of HiAP and One Health, they impose new demands on health systems' data sharing and cross-sectoral collaborations that require standardisation of data formats, material infrastructure, and forms of organising expertise and personnel. These dynamics have a complex "social life" of their own, which makes it difficult to reach conclusions on the state of interoperability in Ghanaian health information system and its HiAP and One-Health agendas. While intersectoral collaboration between central-level organisations still remains limited, local committees have long-established forms of collaborative resource mobilisation in moments of health emergencies. Notably, they do so without recourse to standardised channels of data sharing, but skilfully devise specific adaptations that respond to the needs of the various actors and contextual conditions.

Acknowledgements This work was supported by the German Research Foundation (Grant number DFG TH2432/2-1 "How Democracies Know: Identification Technologies and Quantitative Analyses of Development in Ghana").

References

Abebrese, J. (2011). *Social protection in Ghana. An overview of existing programmes and their prospects and challenges*. FES.

Adaletey, D., Poppe, O., & Braa, J. (2013). Cloud computing for development—Improving the Health Information System in Ghana. In P. Cunningham & M. Cunningham (Eds.), *IST-Africa 2013 Conference Proceedings* (pp. 1–9). IIMC International Information Management Corporation.

Al Dahdah, M., Desgrées Du Loû, A., & Méadel, C. (2015). Mobile health and maternal care: A winning combination for healthcare in the developing world? *Health Policy and Technology, 4*, 225–231.

Awoonor-Williams, J. K., Tadiri, E., & Ratcliffe, H. (n.d.). *Translating research into practice to ensure community engagement for successful primary health care service delivery: The case of CHPS in Ghana*. PHCPI. Retrieved February 22, 2024, from https://www.improvingphc.org/translating-research-practice-ensure-community-engagement-successful-primary-health-care-service-delivery-case-chps-ghana-0

Boadu, R. O. (2004). The use of health information system for planning and decision-making in Ejisu-Juaben District of Ghana. KNUST. Retrieved

February 22, 2024, from https://ir.knust.edu.gh/items/ddc56b58-aff4-43b6-b593-0b6451bbbf2a

Bowker, G., & Star, S. L. (1999). *Sorting things out. Classification and its consequences*. MIT Press.

Carbone, G. (2011). Democratic demands and social policies: The politics of health reform in Ghana. *The Journal of Modern African Studies, 49*(3), 381–408.

CDC. (2023). One health basics. Centers for Disease Control and Prevention. Retrieved February 22, 2024, from https://www.cdc.gov/onehealth/basics/index.html#:~:text=One%20Health%20is%20a%20collaborative,plants%2C%20and%20their%20shared%20environment

GHS. (2023). Information, Monitoring And Evaluation (IME) Department. Retrieved February 22, 2024, from https://ghs.gov.gh/information-monitoring-and-evaluation-ime-department/

Grebe, E. (2015). The evolution of social protection policy in Ghana's 'Fourth Republic': Contributory social insurance reform and limited social assistance for the 'extreme poor' under NPP and NDC governments, 2000–2014. Cape Town: CSSR Working Paper No. 360.

Jolliffe, B., Poppe, O., Adaletey, D., & Braa, J. (2015). Models for online computing in developing countries: Issues and deliberations. *Information Technology for Development, 21*(1), 151–161.

Kwame Adu, G. (2014). Integrating community data into DHIS2. Integrated Community Case Management (iCCM) Evidence Review Symposium, March 3–5, 2014, Accra, Ghana.

Lampland, M., & Star, S. L. (2008). *Standards and their stories. How quantifying, classifying, and formalizing practices shape everyday life*. Cornell University Press.

Light, B., Burgess, J., & Duguay, S. (2018). The walkthrough method: An approach to the study of apps. *New Media & Society, 20*(3), 881–900.

Miscione, G., Staring, K., Østmo, L., & Fossum, K. (2008). The shifting legitimation of an information system: Local, global and large scale. *GlobDev 2008*, 7. http://aisel.aisnet.org/globdev2008/7

NHP. (2020). National Health Policy: Ensuring healthy lives for all. Retrieved February 22, 2024, from https://www.moh.gov.gh/wp-content/uploads/2020/07/NHP_12.07.2020.pdf-13072020-FINAL.pdf

Odei-Lartey, E., Kyerewaa Dwommoh Prah, R., Apraku Anane, E., Danwonno, H., Gyaase, S., Boakye Oppong, F., Afenyadu. G., & Poku Asante, K. (2020). Utilization of the national cluster of district health information system for health service decision-making at the district, subdistrict and community levels in selected districts of the Brong Ahafo region in Ghana. *BMC Health Services Research, 20*(514), 2–15.

Ofosu, A. (2012). DHIMS2 demo using quality health information for decision making. Annual General Conference Medical Superintendents' Group, November 2012. Retrieved February 22, 2024, from https://www.ghanahealthservice.org/ghs-item-details.php?cid=2&scid=55&iid=63

Schinkell, W. (2016). Making climates comparable: Comparison in paleoclimatology. *Social Studies of Science, 46*(3), 374–395.

Star, S. L., & Strauss, A. (1999). Layers of silence, arenas of voice: The ecology of visible and invisible work. *Computer Supported Cooperative Work, 8*, 9–30.

Sulzbach, S., Garshong, B., & Owusu-Banahene, G. (2005). *Evaluating the Effects of the National Health Insurance Act in Ghana*. Bethesda: The Partners for Health Reformplus Project, Abt Associates Inc. Retrieved February 22, 2024, from https://pdf.usaid.gov/pdf_docs/PNADG454.pdf

Sæbø, J., Kwame Kossi, E., Hodne Titlestad, O., Rolland Tohour, R., & Braa, J. (2011). Comparing strategies to integrate health information systems following a data warehouse approach in four countries. *Information Technology for Development, 17*(1), 42–60.

Troeger, J., & Bock, A. (2022). The sociotechnical walkthrough—a methodological approach for platform studies. *Studies in Communication Sciences, 22*(1), 43–52.

WHO. (n.d.). Promoting Health in All Policies and intersectoral action capacities. Retrieved February 22, 2024, from https://www.who.int/activities/promoting-health-in-all-policies-and-intersectoral-action-capacities

CHAPTER 8

Conclusion: Health Data's Social Life

Alena Thiel and Samuel Aniegye Ntewusu

We set out in this book to emphasise the importance of an interdisciplinary reading of knowledge practices in health—whether oral, written, or digital—and the ways in which these practices have intersected with power structures, forces of standardisation, and medical pluralism, at various moments in Ghana's history. Centrally, we were convinced that there remains a need to address the historical gap that exists in the literature on health in Ghana and elsewhere. From the very first attempt at describing and classifying health in Ghana through the production of paper records, to the present efforts at populating digital health registers, the materiality of health registration has undergone important transformations, reflecting at its core shifting political, economic, and socio-medical relations—while simultaneously participating in these transitions.

The contributions in this book have illustrated how the close empirical study of health data practices in the context of medical pluralism

A. Thiel (✉)
Martin-Luther-University Halle-Wittenberg, Halle, Germany
e-mail: alena.thiel@ethnologie.uni-halle.de

S. A. Ntewusu
University of Ghana, Accra, Ghana
e-mail: santewusu@ug.edu.gh

A. Thiel and S. A. Ntewusu (eds.), *The Social Life of Health Data*,
https://doi.org/10.1007/978-981-97-3500-6_8

helps to foreground the coproduction of material infrastructures and knowledge practices, along with their implications for experiences of care, but also the stigma and exclusions associated with certain diagnostic and therapeutic choices. Contributors to this volume explored, in other words, what happens when the force of standardisation "meets" plural medical contexts. They have provided case studies from various health-related fields that show how the standardisation of diagnoses and treatments, often in the context of global funding streams and therapeutic conventions, affects patients and medical professionals, their manoeuvring spaces, and their strategies to access health care, in unexpected ways. For example, while the medicalisation of mental health in Ghana may still carry stigma for those affected, it has allowed mental health professionals to gradually chip away at such harmful societal attitudes. Or, while traditional medical practitioners seem to embrace quantification as a form of professionalisation, they also reject the commercialisation of their practice that this has entailed. In brief, our combination of historical, sociological, and ethnographic approaches has pointed to both mobilisations and demobilisations, and appropriations and resistances, in processes of standardising health.

Our collection of case studies, we hope, contributes a new qualitative perspective to existing studies of management and governance in health systems, and informs ongoing conversations about the regulation of public health services by adding a novel focus on the local adaptations of globally circulating knowledge practices and their standardising forces. In approaching regulatory practices as inherently social, e.g. in Amoni's analysis of the social construction of herbal medical practitioners' professionalism through quantitative evidence-making, we hope to offer a contribution to de-centring the existing literature on public health (information) systems management, and to narrow in on the experiences, contributions, and adaptations of Ghanaian health professionals.

Clashes between global medical standards and care practices in Ghana date far back in history, as evidenced by Oliver Tasin. Tasin's chapter provided important insights into the local adaptations to northern Ghana's environmental conditions and endemic diseases. For Tasin, the link between indigenous approaches to the treatment of diseases and their cosmology is crucial for understanding health and healing in societal perspective. "Control over healing was central to the social and political power exercised by either a healer or traditional leader," Tasin notes. Health, then, did not merely encompass the physiology of the individual body, but "was aimed at promoting societal well-being in order to ensure continuity of the society." Yet to argue that the British administrators simply disrupted this perspective on health and healing when they introduced Western biomedicine would be an oversimplification. As Tasin shows, one needs to consider efforts at the level of the community, the colonial administration, and its transnational, inter-imperial connections, to fully understand the introduction of the colonial health system. While colonial officers initially relied on local medical knowledge and practice for their expansion into northern Ghana, following WWI economic motivations shaped medical interventions, as the north was considered a critical source of human labour for mining, cocoa production, and the development of critical infrastructure such as roads, railways, and security. As noted, health was seen as paramount to British imperial success, and so was the drive to formalise medical knowledge and knowledge production. As a result, the colonial medical approach began to expand biomedical interventions (initially limited to Europeans) onto native populations. This, Tasin shows, not least also had an important transnational dimension, in the form of inter-imperial medical research collaboration and learning. Following this expansion, local knowledge about diseases and healing was silenced, pointing to the strong colonial prejudice against indigenous medical knowledge, and as a potential consequence, the control over or complete erasure of the societal influence of healers.

Samuel Ntewusu's chapter delves into the micro-dynamics of these developments, pointing us to novel insights into the infrastructural bases of expanding biomedical interventions into the colony's remote regions, especially the Northern Territory. From the 1930s, the Medical Field Units (MFUs) were dispatched into Ghana's remote regions to provide essential epidemiological interventions as part of the campaign against trypanosomiasis. Ntewusu and Tasin agree on the economic motivations of expanding biomedical health interventions onto local populations. Adding to Tasin, Ntewusu points us to the enlistment of local populations not only in medical treatment, but also in (elementary) training in diagnostics, surveying (census taking), and crucially, record keeping. This, Ntewusu details, required significant investments in complex hierarchies of staff. Alongside increasing technical specialisation, Ntewusu shows, the campaign saw a proliferation of investments in material infrastructure, including transport infrastructure (with a bias towards bicycles and motorcycles, which were considered more effective in the interior due to a lack of paved roads) and crucially, the development of reporting formats and channels. As disease control measures of the MFU became increasingly complex as a result of the expansion of the campaign into a polyvalent health service, they also increasingly relied on new modes of identifying and targeting specific localities and individuals for intervention, e.g. for the targeted destruction of reservoirs of infection, vaccination, or chemo-prophylaxis. For this reason, the MFU and their survey teams played crucial roles in collecting and transmitting information about diseases.

Yet, besides informing the planning and implementation of various disease control programmes, the MFU's health data production also raises the question of colonial regimes' deployment of metrics (such as censuses and map-making) in the interest of creating and controlling the colonial territory. Especially where the health and mobility of the labour force was concerned, health records seemed to have played an important role in the processes of territorialisation. Ntewusu's analysis reminds us of the power of historical methods to retrace the colonial genealogies of present-day administrative structures, and their potentially continuous haunting[1] through, for example, boundary definitions or the uneven distribution of (medical) infrastructure across the country.

The question of how (colonial) power intersects with and is sustained by health records and interventions is also of relevance to Agyekum's chapter. Ghanaian history shows how mental health legislation in colonial times was intended not to provide care, but rather to police (urban) society. This continues to have implications for access to mental health, as is most clearly visible in the continuous under-investment in mental health facilities and personnel. Building on this observation, Agyekum takes us from the historian's viewpoint into the field of medical anthropology, and thereby, the participation of competing conceptions of mental health and care in treatment and advocacy. Ghanaian mental health professionals' medical practice oscillates between standard case definitions, such as the DSM-5, and cultural perspectives of mental illness rooted in spiritual realms. Yet this creates not only tensions and necessary translations between the different knowledges, but also provides interesting opportunities for change processes. As Agyekum shows, medical anthropology allows us to "connect the local and the global in new ways." While standards can be seen as imposing certain blueprints for intervention, they

[1] Cf. Jordan-Young & Karkazis (2020).

also provide mental health professionals in Ghana with the narrative and argumentative tools to gradually change perceptions.

Standards, in other words, can provide grounds for reading mental health as a "boundary object"[2] that brings together church leaders, school counsellors, and mental health practitioners alike, in the effort to counter the stigmatisation of persons suffering from mental illness and improve access to mental health care. Agyekum provides a hopeful picture of increasing patronage of mental health services over unregulated, and at times harmful spiritual healing practices. His analysis points to significant research desiderata: how will the shift towards medicalised mental health care affect the prevalent stigmatisation of mental illness in Ghanaian society in the future, or in other words, do formal diagnoses reduce or exacerbate societal exclusion? Clearly, future work is needed to trace the effects of mental health professionals' efforts to standardise mental health care.

Similar to Agyekum, Amoni's contribution explores the participation of standardised knowledge practices, here specifically statistical productions, in reshaping attitudes towards care practices. Contrary to Agyekum's fervent support for modernising mental health care, however, Amoni unfolds her analysis of how quantification empowers traditional healing practices. For Amoni, the tensions between biomedicine over traditional medicine since the nineteenth century have important political dimensions. For example, Kwame Nkrumah, the first president of the independent nation of Ghana, actively supported traditional medical practice. But the politics involved in constructing validity around both herbal medical practices and products increasingly demand the production of quantitative forms. Professional associations of herbal practitioners mobilise statistics to both communicate the extent of their membership, and based on this, to push for desired changes in recognising herbal medical practice in Ghana. "The generation of statistics proves to play a significant role in the maintenance and continued existence of the associations," Amoni writes.

Yet again the standardisation of herbal medicine—in the sense of aggregating diverse medical practices under conventionalised quantitative categories—produces complex knowledge encounters. From the perspective of traditional healers, the expectation of health registration for the purpose of quantifying their sector's contributions is experienced as a

[2] Star & Griesemer (1989).

burden. It meets significant opposition as it is seen as "detraditionalising" the practice, through association with commodification. This alignment of traditional healers with social conceptions of health—which as Tasin's chapter noted is rooted in a more holistic understanding of social well-being, besides physiological health, and the moral rejection of (the foregrounding of) monetary compensation—clashes fundamentally with health agendas as defined by Ghanaian state and international organisations, which emphasise a neoliberal path towards development. In view of this, Amoni reminds us to consider the work of efficacy and other standards in setting (at times unrealistic) expectations, and the performative effect of these conventions on the decisions of practitioners. While the drive to improve the safety of herbal medicine in Ghana is crucial, Amoni suggests that a standard rooted in herbal practice itself would provide more fertile grounds to ensure best practices in the sector. Evaluating herbal medicine against standards set in an entirely different field, that is biomedicine, alienates practitioners from the drug regulatory regime, as they "reflect a detachment from the values upon which the practice is anchored."

Where Amoni raises the crucial notion of translation between different sets of standards, and their competing claims to validity, the notion that standards are necessarily localised is also discussed in Senoo-Dogbey, Naab, and Ohene's chapter. Reviewing current practice against international standards, the authors provide an in-depth look at the labour of recording post-exposure interventions to reduce the risk of HBV infection among Ghanaian healthcare workers. Adopting a public health perspective, the authors show how standardisation of reporting on exposure patterns, and the active surveillance of HBV in health facilities, are of crucial importance for the uptake of preventive interventions, PEP management, and ultimately, the use of information for decision-making. At the same time, their analysis illustrates how suboptimal adherence to standard precaution protocols, poor exposure reporting, and PEP management practices are linked to multiple infrastructural but also behavioural challenges beyond the reporting chain. All this serves as a critical reminder about the extensive labour required to not only define and communicate standards in concrete guidelines and protocols, but also to realise them materially, logistically, and in terms of behavioural changes. While standardisation can contribute to awareness-building, as Agyekum shows for the case of mental health advocacy, if there is a continued underinvestment in clinical infrastructure and provision of supplies, the impact of awareness-raising remains unsurprisingly limited.

Reporting standards alone also fail to provide promised gains in efficiency and rationalisation if health practitioners are continuously forced to adapt their practices to breakdowns and other infrastructural tensions, such as missing devices. This is illustrated in the implementation of digital health records described in the book's final empirical chapter. Focusing on the empirics of the production and circulation of digital health data allows us to understand how notions of efficiency, transparency, and accountability in health care datafication do not automatically facilitate better care. As we have seen in the preceding chapters, they require significant labour to populate registers, and forms of organisation that determine avenues of database access. Scholars have further raised neoliberal critiques regarding the infrastructure's application in the surveillance of healthcare providers, while putting new demands on health workers to populate the digital registers. While larger initiatives promote digital tools with the promise of interoperability across societal sectors, in practice inter-agency collaboration requires significant investments in relationship-building, and often relies on analogue tools and communication channels to complement the work of the digital health register.

Throughout all case studies in this book, one theme reverberated. Health registers have a complex "social life," as do culturally embedded practices of healing and care. The authors contributing to this book have shown the skillful adaptations to (globally) circulating standards in the moment of their encounter with medical pluralism. We further highlight the need to decentre our view and move closer to the social construction of health, through practices of recording medical knowledge. The historical method in particular points us to the need to study processes of knowledge production, while the anthropological and sociological perspectives in this book uncovered their diverse impacts on plural medical practices.

In this concluding remark, we also want to point a way forward for research and policy by proposing a comprehensive documentation of multiple forms of health and health documentation. This is considered necessary in providing a holistic view of datafication and standardisation of health in Ghana. The chapters in this book directly or indirectly point to this need. For example, in developing "Policy Guidelines on Traditional Medicine Development" (2005), the Ghanaian Ministry of Health indicated that "there is no single document that coordinates the general policy direction of government in the area of traditional medicine."[3] This book could not agree more with the above as regards the need for policy direction, and for the framework of government to provide an across-the-board approach, involving different health actors, to developing a comprehensive data system that will guide health practice and delivery in Ghana.

References

Jordan-Young, R., & Karkazis, K. (2020). Sensing race as a ghost variable in science, technology, and medicine. *Science, Technology, and Human Values, 45*(5), 763–778.

Ministry of Health. (2005). Policy Guidelines on Traditional Medicine Development. https://www.moh.gov.gh/wp-content/uploads/2016/02/TRADITIONAL-MEDICINE-POLICY.pdf

Star, S., & Griesemer, J. (1989). Institutional ecology, 'translations' and boundary objects: Amateurs and Professionals in Berkeley's museum of vertebrate zoology, 1907–39. *Social Studies of Science, 19*(3), 387–420.

[3] Ministry of Health (2005).

Index

A. Thiel and S. A. Ntewusu (eds.), *The Social Life of Health Data*,
https://doi.org/10.1007/978-981-97-3500-6

The manufacturer's authorised representative in the EU is Springer Nature Customer Service Centre GmbH, Europaplatz 3, 69115 Heidelberg, Germany. If you have any concerns regarding our products, please contact ProductSafety@springernature.com

Printed and bound by CPI Group (UK) Ltd, Croydon, CR0 4YY
30/09/2026
02225286-0001